Human Factors and Ergonomics in Health and Social Care

An Applied Approach

Mark Sujan, Laura Pickup,
Helen Vosper and Ken Catchpole

Class Professional Publishing have made every effort to ensure that the information, tables, drawings and diagrams contained in this book are accurate at the time of publication. The book cannot always contain all the information necessary for determining appropriate care and cannot address all individual situations; therefore, individuals using the book must ensure they have the appropriate knowledge and skills to enable suitable interpretation. Class Professional Publishing do not guarantee, and accept no legal liability of whatever nature arising from, or connected to, the accuracy, reliability, currency or completeness of the content of *Human Factors and Ergonomics in Health and Social Care – An Applied Approach*. Users must always be aware that such innovations or alterations after the date of publication may not be incorporated in the content. Please note, however, that Class Professional Publishing assume no responsibility whatsoever for the content of external resources in the text or accompanying online materials.

Text © Mark Sujan, Laura Pickup, Helen Vosper, Ken Catchpole 2025

All rights reserved. Without limiting the rights under copyright reserved above, no part of this publication may be reproduced, stored in or introduced into a retrieval system, or transmitted, in any form or by any means (electronic, mechanical, photocopying, recording or otherwise) without the prior written permission of the publisher of this book.

The information presented in this book is accurate and current to the best of the authors' knowledge. The authors and publisher, however, make no guarantee as to, and assume no responsibility for, the correctness, sufficiency or completeness of such information or recommendation.

Printing history
This edition first published in 2025.

The authors and publisher welcome feedback from the users of this book. Please contact the publisher:

Class Professional Publishing,
The Exchange, Express Park, Bristol Road, Bridgwater TA6 4RR
Telephone: 01278 472 800
Email: info@class.co.uk
Website: www.classprofessional.co.uk

Class Professional Publishing is an imprint of Class Publishing Ltd
A CIP catalogue record for this book is available from the British Library

Paperback ISBN: 9781801610933
ePub ISBN: 9781801610940
ePDF ISBN: 9781801610957

Cover design by Nicky Borowiec
Designed and typeset by PHi Business Solutions
Printed in the UK by Hobbs

This book is printed on paper from responsible sources. Refer to local recycling guidance on disposal of this book.

Product safety information can be found at https://www.classprofessional.co.uk/terms-of-use/gpsr-statement/

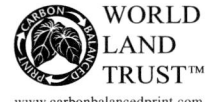

In this first-of-a-kind book, four authors with solid pedigrees in practice and research in the field have come together to help explain what human factors and ergonomics (HF/E) is and how to do it. The book covers the key topics that comprise HF/E in practice, supporting the Healthcare Learning Pathway of the Chartered Institute of Ergonomics and Human Factors, and building in the professional competencies for practitioners. The result is a practical and readable book that will help readers upskill to membership of the CIEHF, so that they can help integrate HF/E in practice in their own organisation to help improve system performance and human well-being.

Steven Shorrock, co-editor of *Human Factors and Ergonomics in Practice*, Adjunct Associate Professor, University of the Sunshine Coast, Australia.

This great 'how-to' book is an excellent reference for patient safety leaders and clinicians interested in applying human factors principles in their operational safety work. It is also valuable for human factors professionals working in the healthcare domain. The structure of the book makes it easy to use with chapters covering the basic concepts of safety, which are all made operationally relevant and applied to practice.

Rollin J. 'Terry' Fairbanks, Senior Vice President, Chief Quality and Safety Officer, MedStar Health.

At last, a book about Human Factors & Ergonomics (HF/E) in healthcare written by chartered professionals who are highly experienced in related research, education, and practice and have a particular focus on patient safety. This fantastic offering makes a huge contribution to outlining both foundational and more advanced HF/E principles, concepts and methods that healthcare leaders, practitioners, educators, scientists, risk, safety and improvement advisors and many others can readily apply. Importantly, this timely contribution lays all of this out in a very readable and accessible fashion, with the welcome bonus that it provides much-needed practical guidance on the purpose and approach of HF/E which is sometimes misunderstood in healthcare. This is a must-read for everyone with a strong interest in improving organisational performance and the wellbeing of people who work in, and use, healthcare services.

Paul Bowie, Programme Director (Safety & Improvement), NHS Education for Scotland.

Contents

	About the Authors	ix
	Foreword	xi
	Preface	xiii
1.	**Introduction**	**1**
	Human Factors and Ergonomics for Improving Systems	1
	What Does HF/E Mean in the Context of Health and Social Care?	2
	A Systems Approach	4
	The Systems Engineering Initiative for Patient Safety	5
	Designing Improvement Interventions in Different Types of Systems	10
	How Do We Do HF/E?	13
	Chapter Summary	15
	CIEHF HF/E Competencies	16
	References	16
2.	**The Organisation**	**17**
	Introduction: Understanding and Shaping the Role of Your Organisation in Defining the Work Context	17
	Organisational Culture and Safety Culture	20
	What Does a Positive Safety Culture Look Like?	23
	Measuring Performance	27
	Health and Social Care Safety Culture Discussion Cards	29
	Performance-Influencing Factors Relating to Organisational Culture	31
	Organisational Resilience	33
	Just Culture	34
	Chapter Summary	35
	CIEHF HF/E Competencies	35
	References	35
3.	**Tasks**	**37**
	Introduction: Designing Tasks for Human Performance	37
	Task Types	39
	Task Selection	39
	Studying Clinical Work Using Task Analysis	40

Contents

Identifying Vulnerabilities in Clinical Tasks Using Structured Human Failure Analysis	45
Intervention Selection	51
Implementation and Monitoring	53
Chapter Summary	53
CIEHF HF/E Competencies	53
References	54

4. The People — 55

Introduction: Understanding the Capabilities of the People Working Within Your System	55
Match of Human Capabilities to Tasks	56
Performance-Influencing Factors	58
Designing to Meet Human Characteristics – Inclusive Design	65
Designing for Inclusion	66
Practical Methods for Capturing User Experience and Requirements	69
Chapter Summary	71
CIEHF HF/E Competencies	72
References	72

5. Teamwork and Non-Technical Skills — 75

Introduction: Understanding the Social, Cognitive and Personal Skills that Enable People to Perform Tasks in the Work Environment	75
Teamwork in Health and Social Care	77
The Seven Cs Model	79
TeamSTEPPS	80
Non-Technical Skills Frameworks	80
Cognition, Situation Awareness, Sense Making and Decision Making	82
Other Decision-Making Models	85
Delivery	86
Words of Caution	86
Chapter Summary	88
CIEHF HF/E Competencies	88
References	88

6. The Environment — 91

Introduction: Understanding the Context Provided by the Environment and Its Impact on People	91
Is the Environment Fit for Purpose?	92
Physical Fit Within an Environment	93
Layout of the Environment	96
Human Performance Relative to the Environment	101

The Impact of Healthcare Environments on Decision Making	107
Environment and Potential to Influence Well-Being	109
Chapter Summary	110
CIEHF HF/E Competencies	110
References	111

7. Tools and Technologies — 113

- Introduction: Understanding How the Tools We Use Influence How We Work and Deliver Care — 113
- Basic Technology Considerations — 114
- Regulatory Approaches — 120
- Tools and Technology Design Examples — 123
- Chapter Summary — 126
- CIEHF HF/E Competencies — 126
- References — 126

8. Applying Human Factors/Ergonomics to Understanding Outcomes — 129

- Introduction: What Matters and How Do We Know How We Are Doing? — 129
- Identifying Different Types of Outcomes in a Specific Context — 130
- Impact of Interactions on Outcomes — 132
- Measurement and Monitoring of Outcomes — 133
- Measurement Futures — 136
- Chapter Summary — 136
- CIEHF HF/E Competencies — 137
- References — 137

9. Organisational Learning — 139

- Introduction: Improving Systems Through Learning from Experience — 139
- Organisational Learning in Healthcare — 140
- Why Are Health and Social Care Organisations Not Learning? — 142
- A New Outlook for Organisational Learning — 143
- A Systems-Based Framework for Organisational Learning: Achieving Sustainable Change — 144
- The Patient Safety Incident Response Framework — 146
- Chapter Summary — 150
- CIEHF HF/E Competencies — 150
- References — 150

10. Equality, Diversity and Inclusion — 153

- Introduction: Designing Health and Social Care to Meet Diverse Needs — 153
- Why Are Many Health and Care Systems Not Inclusive? — 155
- Protected Characteristics Are Person Factors — 157

Contents

Taking a Systems Approach to Highlight EDI Issues	159
Participation as a Mechanism for Delivering Equality, Diversity and Inclusion	160
What Might Participatory HF/E Look Like in Health and Social Care?	162
ISO 27500 (The Human Centred Organization)	163
Chapter Summary	165
CIEHF HF/E Competencies	165
References	165

11. Human Factors Integration — **167**

Introduction: Developing Processes for Embedding and Evidencing Human Factors/Ergonomics	167
Human Factors Integration Principles	168
Why is Human Factors Integration Necessary for Health and Social Care?	170
What Could Human Factors Integration Look Like in Health and Social Care?	171
What Might We Need to Consider to Develop a Human Factors Integration Strategy?	173
Chapter Summary	176
CIEHF HF/E Competencies	176
References	177

12. Epilogue: The Future of Human Factors/Ergonomics in Health and Social Care — **179**

Introduction	179
The Evolving Landscape of Health and Social Care	180
The Educational Landscape for HF/E in Health and Social Care	181
Achieving Sustainable Change	184

Index — 185

About the Authors

Mark Sujan is Professor of Safety Science at the University of York and a Senior Investigation Science Educator at the Health Services Safety Investigations Body (HSSIB). He is a Chartered Ergonomist (C.ErgHF) and Managing Director of Human Factors Everywhere. The company provides ergonomics input to applied research projects and offers consultancy and training in ergonomics across a range of safety-critical industries. Mark is a Trustee of the Chartered Institute of Ergonomics and Human Factors, and he leads the Institute's special interest group on Digital Health & Artificial Intelligence.

Laura Pickup is the Head of Human Factors at the University Hospitals Bristol and Weston. She is a Chartered Ergonomist (C.ErgHF) and a Director of LP Human Factors, which provides human factors input for healthcare investigations, training and applied research in healthcare. Laura works across an NHS Trust and independently to understand and address patient safety issues. She has considerable experience in the development of human factors methods, which inform physical and cognitive work and device design.

Helen Vosper is the Lead for Patient Safety at the University of Aberdeen and a Senior Investigation Science Educator at the HSSIB. She is also a Scientific Advisor in Human Factors and Patient Safety at NHS Education for Scotland. She is a Chartered Ergonomist (C.ErgHF) and a Principal Fellow Advance HE (PFHEA).

Ken Catchpole is the SmartState Endowed Chair in Clinical Practice and Human Factors at the Medical University of South Carolina. He is a clinically embedded research practitioner, who has been applying human factors principles to improve safety and performance in acute care since 2003. He has authored over 100 peer-reviewed journal articles relating to patient safety and human factors, while working alongside clinicians at the front line to understand everyday challenges and to address a broad range of reliability, safety and performance concerns from a human-centred perspective. Ken is a Registered Member of the Chartered Institute of Ergonomics and Human Factors (MCIEHF).

Foreword

There is an ever-growing demand for human factors knowledge in health and social care. This has created an appetite for clinicians, patient safety professionals and even some qualified human factors professionals, entering healthcare for the first time, to understand the practical application of our scientific discipline in the clinical and care environment.

This book offers an excellent resource for those looking to increase the breadth of their human factors skills, providing examples to illustrate typical health and social care issues. The book has framed itself around the fundamental sociotechnical systems principle of human factors, using the well-known SEIPS framework (Systems Engineering Initiative for Patient Safety) to describe where and how human factors can be considered irrespective of the care setting. The handbook style aims to guide the reader to consider their own work or care setting and to be creative in how practically they can use the principles or concepts described. This is an excellent resource for those new to the field or looking to consolidate their existing human factors education.

Each chapter seeks to answer a set of questions by providing examples and sharing the authors' cumulative 50 years of experience working in the area of health and social care. They have helpfully mapped the content to the current health and social care learning pathway and to competencies that have been outlined by the Chartered Institute of Ergonomics and Human Factors (CIEHF). This guides the reader to understand where and how to develop their own human factors journey and to consider the different levels of membership and accreditation that they may wish to consider undertaking to establish their own capability and professional skills in this discipline.

As the current President of the CIEHF I welcome this pragmatic book, which can help health and social care to build the capacity to deliver human factors. This will in turn support bringing healthcare in line with other industries where the scientific discipline and professional practice of human factors have actively contributed to improvements in safety and performance.

Mark Young, President, CIEHF

Preface

NHS England set out a vision for patient safety in the NHS Patient Safety Strategy. This includes a focus on education and training, with the aspiration to educate patient safety specialists, who can provide leadership with a systems focus based on insights from human factors and ergonomics (HF/E) and safety science. The Chartered Institute of Ergonomics and Human Factors (CIEHF) maintains a set of professional competencies for human factors specialists. This book intends to operationalise these and make them accessible to a wider audience in health and social care, in line with the vision for education and training set out in the NHS Patient Safety Strategy.

In July 2021, CIEHF launched the Healthcare Learning Pathway in collaboration with its partners at Loughborough University, Robert Gordon University, NHS Education for Scotland and Human Factors Everywhere, and in partnership with Health Education England and the Royal College of Nursing. The Healthcare Learning Pathway takes students on a journey from thinking differently about systems and safety, to the scientific background underpinning the discipline, and on to integrating HF/E in practice. The Healthcare Learning Pathway is organised into three levels: Level 1 is an accredited one-hour online course, introducing students to the ways in which HF/E can contribute to improving health and social care work; Level 2 provides a certificate in HF/E science, covering aspects such as systems, the analysis of tasks and processes, the design of interfaces and the structure and processes of organisational learning; Level 3 offers a route to an accredited qualification (such as TechCIEHF), achieved through one-to-one learning with a CIEHF specialist as mentor to support students with the application of HF/E in their practice.

This book complements the Healthcare Learning Pathway and is intended as a practical resource for students. The book aims to provide well-founded, practical guidance to those responsible for leading and implementing HF/E programmes and interventions in health and social care. The book is structured around the different elements of a work system, where practitioners might place their focus. For each element, the nature of issues that are frequently addressed is given, followed by a characterisation of available HF/E methods and approaches. Where appropriate and feasible, we describe in more detail a selection of representative and important HF/E methods and approaches using a practical example. This will help guide practitioners through the many opportunities for HF/E interventions and the wide range of methods to choose from. Each chapter concludes with a list of CIEHF professional competencies addressed. This can help the readers who are considering an application for technical specialist or registered member of CIEHF. As part of the application form, the applicant needs to indicate their level of expertise of the CIEHF

Preface

professional competencies and support this with evidence, such as project reports. The overview of the CIEHF professional competencies at the end of each chapter can help the reader to think about the kinds of evidence that might be appropriate to demonstrate different competencies. To note, the CIEHF professional competencies are not static and are undergoing regular review. However, while the number of competencies and their wording might change, the content overall is not expected to change significantly, and the list of competencies used in the book (2023/2024) is likely to remain a good guide.

The book is intended to be read sequentially, but readers can also jump to chapters of particular relevance to their interest. It is advisable to start with the Introduction (Chapter 1), as this provides an overview of HF/E and the systems approach used in the book. The following chapters (Chapter 2–7) discuss the different elements of a work system. If you are interested in a specific aspect, for example the physical environment, you could prioritise the relevant chapter accordingly. Chapter 8 looks at outcomes based on the systems perspective and relates outcomes back to interactions of the elements of the work system. The remaining chapters (Chapters 9–11) build on the systems perspective introduced in the first part of the book and cover further topics on organisational learning, equality, diversity and inclusion, as well as how to integrate and embed HF/E. The final chapter (chapter 12) considers the future, challenges and how to build your role in human factors within health and social care.

The CIEHF received its Royal Charter in 2014 to recognise the uniqueness and value of the scientific discipline and the pre-eminent role of the Institute in representing both the discipline and the profession in the UK. This includes the protected status of 'Chartered Ergonomist and Human Factors Specialist', with the post-nominal C.ErgHF, awarded to practising Registered Members and Fellows who are among a group of elite professionals working at a world-class level.

We would like to thank Dr Noorzaman Rashid for his enthusiasm and encouragement towards this book.

Mark Sujan
Laura Pickup
Helen Vosper
Ken Catchpole

CHAPTER 1

Introduction

Chapter Objectives and Learning Outcomes

- To explain what human factors/ergonomics (HF/E) and a systems approach are.
- To understand what to look at within a healthcare work system.
- To be familiar with how HF/E approaches the improvement of system outcomes.
- To understand how HF/E practitioners achieve their work.

Human Factors and Ergonomics for Improving Systems

Human factors and ergonomics (HF/E) help with an understanding of health and social care systems and improve outcomes, such as patient safety and staff well-being. This book can be used by anyone looking to improve such outcomes within the fields of health and social care. We recognise that many readers may have some existing knowledge of HF/E principles and methods. The book aims to provide a sense check of any existing knowledge and to support the practical application of HF/E, while signposting further resources for deeper study. Each of the chapters focuses on a specific element of the work system. The chapters explore how HF/E can help understand the interactions between these elements of a work system. HF/E can become a way of thinking about patient safety and other concerns by understanding how the system creates the opportunity for successful or unsuccessful work and delivery of care.

This chapter introduces the basic principles of HF/E and unpacks the individual elements to be considered in the context of a work system. This covers the ways in which different elements may influence outcomes relating to safety, efficiency and well-being, and HF/E aims to design safety into a system (see Box 1.1 for an example).

BOX 1.1 An example of an HF/E approach to organisational change

A large Trust wished to procure beds that were suitable for all areas of the hospital. The HF/E support was requested to support the Trust's decision making to ensure that the procurement contract that was agreed would safeguard the safety of patients and staff, while also providing the best financial arrangement for the Trust.

A full scoping of the clinical areas and the patients cared for was completed to identify the intended users of the beds, which included adult and paediatric patients, clinical staff, cleaners and porters, to understand the key activities they would be required to complete with the beds and the preferred features of the beds that would support those activities. The subsequent evaluation of the beds to support these activities was based on the ability for them to guarantee the safety of staff and patients and the associated efficiency of the activities. Analysis of the environments in which the beds were intended to be used and other equipment likely to interact with the beds ensured a complete insight of the properties to be considered as essential or desirable in the beds to be procured by the Trust. Checks of the size of doorways, lifts and floor space ensured that any bed could be moved between clinical areas. Rarely is healthcare equipment used alone, and beds were considered key to supporting monitors, drip stands or mattresses, all of which need to fit securely and easily.

Different companies provided a range of different bed products, including specific beds for paediatrics and bariatric patients. Ultimately, the final decision was made following an evaluation of all relevant types of bed, through a trial (product evaluation) with representative user groups to evaluate how well each product could support the activities required. There were just two companies able to support all types of beds required, with the final decision made based on the contract agreed to ensure the maintenance and reliability of all stock required.

What Does HF/E Mean in the Context of Health and Social Care

The acronym HF/E reflects both human factors and ergonomics, which are used interchangeably, as they have the same aims. These are defined by the International Ergonomics Association as follows:

> *Human factors is concerned with the understanding of* **interactions among humans and other elements of a system**. *It's the profession that applies theory, principles, data and methods to* **design** *to optimise* **human well-being** *and overall* **system performance**. *Practitioners contribute to the design and evaluation of tasks, jobs, products, environments and systems to make them compatible with the needs, abilities and limitations of people.*

The term 'system' is frequently used in the field of HF/E and has an intuitive meaning to most people, but this may not be the same meaning. In healthcare, the term system may refer to a purely technical system in the form of a piece of equipment. For example, the patient's bed and the interaction between the technical components of the bed form a distinct technical system. As an HF/E practitioner we would want to understand the safety, functionality and reliability of the bed in the intended clinical setting and with the people likely to interact with the bed. This extends the boundary of the system, from just the technical elements within the bed to how the bed functions in the context of the necessary environment to support the tasks that need to be completed to deliver everyday patient care, or emergency interventions. This would be regarded as a sociotechnical system. Consider an unstable patient being transferred to intensive care. Can we be sure that the bed can fit between all doors, can be moved easily without injuring those transporting the patient, can enable emergency care if required in transit, and can support all necessary monitoring and medical devices required by the patient? How easily can staff clean and maintain the bed to ensure a high level of performance based on its design and use? A hospital bed may seem to be a basic requirement for every hospital. Yet, this single piece of equipment may fundamentally influence the safety of the patient transfer and the ability of support staff to deliver emergency treatment if required in transit, may avoid staff injury and ensure the reliability and therefore availability of beds to which patients may be admitted. The compatibility of the humble hospital bed, procured by an organisation, may potentially influence patient safety, hospital efficiency and staff sickness and absence.

When organisations start to look at and understand how people function or accommodate the equipment and environments they work within, to fulfil the tasks required, they start to understand how healthcare systems really achieve their safety and performance. This is the fundamental approach adopted by HF/E to consider how systems interact and how work is really done. HF/E therefore applies the principles of design to optimise the equipment, environments and tasks to make it easier for people and organisations to do the right thing efficiently, make it hard to do the wrong thing and, ideally, make it impossible to do anything that may cause harm. HF/E places people at the centre of the system and designs the system to support the capabilities and constraints associated with people in the system.

HF/E has been described as having twin aims, which are not mutually exclusive (see Figure 1.1) (Wilson and Corlett, 1995). Any HF/E improvement or intervention should consider the well-being of people in the system to be directly related to the safety, efficiency and cost-effectiveness of an organisation. For example, the preservation of an effective break system for staff may enhance the performance of clinical tasks and reduce injury, and can influence time lost to delays in clinical tasks, sickness and absence of staff, which may incur the cost of hiring agency staff. Presenting data to an organisation, which represents the cost associated with a safety concern, can be an effective approach to proposing the value of an HF/E approach and designing systems to balance safety and well-being alongside system performance and efficiency goals.

HF/E can be used to consider any type of system, simple or complex, technical or sociotechnical. It would be wise to be clear about the boundary of the system that is the focus of any safety improvement. This will give you clarity about its limitations and help you to ensure a realistic timeframe to your work.

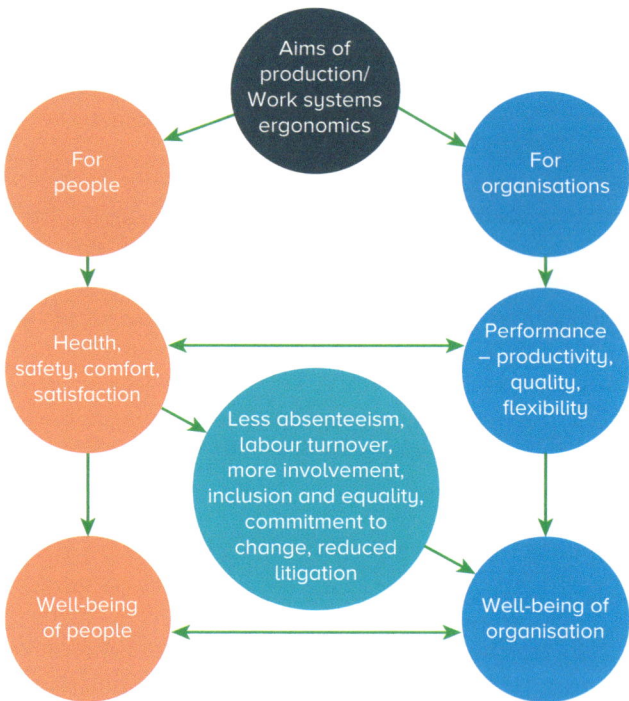

FIGURE 1.1 Twin aims of HF/E.
Source: Based on Wilson and Corlett, 1995.

A Systems Approach

'A systems approach' is a term often associated with HF/E. A system consists of a number of distinct elements, which work together to achieve a common goal. It is widely acknowledged that there is a need to understand the individual elements of a system, while simultaneously recognising that the interaction between the individual elements is dynamic and the value of the whole system is greater than the sum of the parts (Wilson, 2014). A systems approach considers how the elements of the system do, or could, interact with each other and influence a particular outcome.

The fundamental misunderstanding that safety in health and social care systems, or any other safety-related system, might be enhanced as long as we identify the 'bad apples' among staff, is finally starting to be recognised. A single element, unless in the simplest system, is rarely found as the 'cause' of an incident or safety issue. For example, the skill set of the staff available in a unit, at any single moment, will be influenced by the organisation's approach to the recruitment and sustainability of staff, the competence training programmes provided, the rostering of staff, and acknowledgement of the consistent set of skills required to enable a unit to function. The performance of staff within a unit may need to compensate for other elements in the system. Understanding which element of the system is compensating more than another needs to be teased out to recognise key influences on the current functionality of the whole system. The ability to achieve this understanding and avoid 'bad apple'-thinking requires organisational processes to reflect a systems approach (Russ et al., 2013). Do risk assessments consider the whole system; do procedures and policies consider the typical context and environment where they are used; does incident reporting or investigation move beyond just focusing on the actions of frontline staff? To achieve effective integration of HF/E into health and social care systems, a systems approach must inform the design of organisational processes, environments, equipment and documentation.

Adopting a systems approach to the design of health and social care systems can provide a framework to acknowledge that although staff are often involved in the last interaction prior to an incident, generally their actions and behaviour are the product of influences from the whole work system. This can also change the language used when looking at unintended or undesirable outcomes, where a single 'cause' may not be evident, but a systems approach can provide evidence of the interaction of contributory factors. Identification of contributory factors provides a rich source of information and understanding of where to target improvement resources.

Understanding how a system works is achieved by taking the time to look at the elements of a system and how they typically interact with each other. This can reveal which elements are most influential or likely to contribute to particular outcomes, which elements are most dependent upon others, and which elements may be compensating for the insufficiencies of other elements.

The Systems Engineering Initiative for Patient Safety

Adopting a systems approach can be made easier to apply with a framework from which to begin work, as we all need a map to navigate unfamiliar terrains. There are many frameworks used by HF/E practitioners to represent system design. One specifically developed for healthcare contexts is the Systems Engineering Initiative for Patient Safety (SEIPS) (Carayon et al., 2020; Holden and Carayon, 2021; Holden et al., 2013) (Figure 1.2).

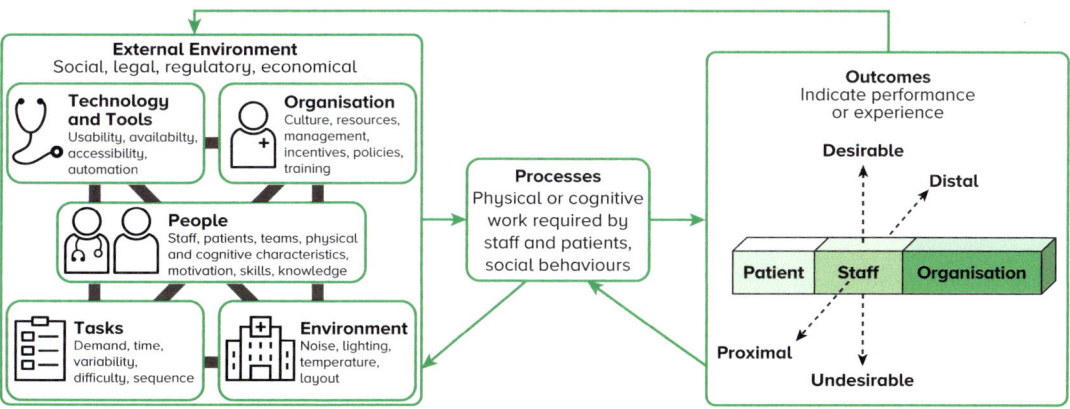

FIGURE 1.2 Systems Engineering Initiative for Patient Safety (SEIPS).

SEIPS was developed early in 2000 to integrate concepts from engineering, HF/E and Donabedian's model for evaluating the quality of care (Donabedian, 1988). SEIPS is a model that provides a way to consider what a particular work system looks like (left side of the model) in the context of where care is delivered, which influences the clinician's work and patient care (middle of the model) and subsequently impacts upon the outcome for the patient, staff and organisation (right side of the model). Put simply, the model can focus relevant questions to understand what and who does the work, how and where work and care happen and what impact all of these factors have upon the effectiveness and experience of patients, staff and healthcare organisations.

The SEIPS model emphasises feedback loops as a feature of how dynamic systems monitor, respond to and adapt to system outcomes. The dynamic and adaptive properties required of healthcare systems are a fundamental strength, and healthcare is considered to be a complex sociotechnical system. The adaptations or trade-offs made by staff or by the wider system may signal stress and strain in the system, which may influence the ability to deliver a service. Adaptations may also lead to emergent properties within a system, which may not all be predictable or advantageous, with some having a disproportionate impact on a patient's care compared to what might appear a relatively minor adaptation. For example, the procurement of a technical system that does not interact with an existing system may require staff to adapt and duplicate entries or delay inputting patient information. Multiple entries of similar information increase the chance of an entry being incorrectly made, and can increase staff workload, which staff compensate for by not taking breaks. This may lead to reduced reliability in patient records, increased risk of staff fatigue and increased stress, which all have the potential to influence patient safety.

SEIPS suggests two perspectives to the outcome produced by the system based on a perspective of time. Typically in healthcare we will consider success or the safety of patients relative to outcomes immediate or 'proximal' to their care, such as, for example, a missed clinical treatment. The implication of the outcome 'distal' to the time when care was delivered (for example, steady loss of functional independence for a patient) may not be directly linked to an episode of care. The implication of how we consider the impact or cost of safety issues in healthcare is usually consideration of the more immediate and visible impacts.

We use SEIPS throughout the book to provide a helpful visualisation of how the work system (the elements within the system, people, equipment, environment, tasks and the organisation) influences the safety of the processes that are necessary to care for or manage a patient within a specific area of health and social care (Box 1.2 and Table 1.1).

We can use SEIPS to guide our interrogation of the system and to look retrospectively at an undesirable outcome. The example of returned blood results in Table 1.1 uses SEIPS to consider the contributory system factors that influenced the failure in the return of a blood sample. SEIPS can become a useful tool or a way of thinking about how the system can be examined and unpicked to identify the what, who, how and

BOX 1.2 Receiving blood results

Several incidents in the failure of the return of blood samples to GPs were not identified for over twelve months. These incidents were reviewed to gain an understanding of how the system prevented the reliable return of the results and an immediate recognition in the failure of the system.

The return of blood test results to a primary care setting requires interaction and communication across multiple technical systems and healthcare settings. Once a test is completed in a hospital setting, the sample may be processed within an external laboratory; the results, once processed, will be communicated through IT systems.

Test results are received and processed by primary care administrative staff. Results that suggest abnormalities or the need for a medical review must be identified, prioritised and the relevant staff and patients informed.

TABLE 1.1 Analysis of receiving blood results using SEIPS

Work system	Prompt	How it applies to receiving blood results
Task	What is being done?	How the transfer of information is completed between different systems; prompts and assurances in the need to look for incoming results; identifying and interpreting results that require additional action; recognising failure of results to return.
Tool/technology	What is being used?	The interaction of multiple technical systems; how software and interface design support tasks; the completeness in the recording and logging of outgoing and incoming results.
Environment	Where is it being done?	Communication of information: across multiple organisations and distributed locations (healthcare organisation and patient homes). Attention and interpretation of information: noisy, distracting work environments with competing tasks.
People	Who influences it?	The patient might be proactive if informed of when to expect results. Staff checking test results routinely or as patient attends an appointment.

(*continued*)

TABLE 1.1 (*continued*)

Work system	Prompt	How it applies to receiving blood results
Organisation	How is it being completed?	Procurement of technical systems with the capability to alert failure in the return of results; interface design to identify failure in the return of results; proactive assessment of the risks and complexities of technical communication systems; the impact of software updates or changes in system configuration or staff resources on the reliability of result handling.
External	What outside of the organisation may be of influence?	The national guidance and evaluation of technical systems, which NHS providers can procure. The national or international standards for testing that systems are fit for purpose and minimise use error and failure.
Process	Return of blood result	How might the following be influenced: recorded analysis of blood samples; transfer of blood results; recognition of the arrival of results; interpretation of results and communication of results to patients; alert for failure of results to return.
Outcome	Proximal and distal impact upon patients, staff and healthcare organisations	Accurate and timely return of all test results aligned to the correct patient. For the patient this may impact the timing of their treatment or diagnosis; clinically this may influence the ability to minimise hospitalisation or treatment; and for staff an effective work system may reduce the stress and workload associated with ensuring all test results are managed efficiently and effectively.

where that influence the way work and care happens. This 'way of thinking' is how HF/E intends to inform healthcare's goal to improve patient safety and experience, as well as staff well-being. HF/E provides a well-established approach to view the person as just one part of the system, with the design of the system directly influencing the way work is done and outcomes are achieved.

HF/E strives to influence all aspects of the system from the design of tasks and processes, the equipment, and the work environment, to reflect the physical and cognitive capabilities and limitations, preferences and expectancies of the people involved. A core aim of HF/E is to make it easier for people to do the right thing, hard for them to do the wrong thing and, ideally, impossible for them to cause harm.

Chapter 1 Introduction

SEIPS can also be used proactively to inform a risk assessment or the planning of new services and even physical spaces (Table 1.2). For example, the development of a new theatre suite or intensive care unit could consider the system to ensure all users are consulted to understand the tasks they complete, the environment required and the equipment likely to be used, stored and transferred between different healthcare procedures and processes.

TABLE 1.2 SEIPS as a framework to guide the design or evaluation of a new workplace

Work system	Prompt	How it applies to the design of a new system
Task	What is being done?	What are the lighting requirements, power supplies, temperature relevant to tasks? What are the physical and cognitive properties of the tasks? How do tasks come together to deliver a specific function, and can the environment and equipment support this?
Tool/ technology	What is being used?	How will equipment and tools be stored, moved and accommodated within clinical spaces? Which equipment interacts to support particular tasks? Can the safety of tasks be supported to minimise use error or avoid known safety issues through the tools and technology?
Environment	Where is it being done?	How can the environment enhance the physical and cognitive requirements of the tasks required? Will lighting, temperature or noise have an impact on tasks and human performance, such as safety-critical communication or decision making? How will storage of all equipment and medication meet policies and practical requirements, based on an understanding of tasks?
People	Who influences it?	What are the physical characteristics of the users; can the shortest staff reach lights or drug cupboards; can the tallest staff read computer screens or avoid banging their head on low hanging infrastructure?
Organisation	How is it being completed?	How will breaks be accommodated? Are rest areas compatible to the number of staff; do they support napping ; do they provide access to food and drink at any time of day?
External	What outside of the organisation may be of influence?	National guidance on design, regulatory requirements, funding allocated.

(continued)

TABLE 1.2 *(continued)*

Work system	Prompt	How it applies to the design of a new system
Process	Admission to the clinical area Delivery of care Transfer to other clinical settings	How might the following be influenced: IT systems used to admit, check or transfer patient information; layout, space and flow between key tasks within and across interrelated clinical areas and with staff and patient group.
Outcome	Proximal and distal impact upon patients, staff and healthcare organisations	Is the environment designed to support the safe and efficient delivery of care? Is there effective interaction across different healthcare processes and environments? Is it easy and safe for all staff roles to provide care? Is there effective and efficient management of patient conditions? Staff well-being and job satisfaction should increase; there should be a decrease in recovery time for patients and a minimising of the risk of harm.

Designing Improvement Interventions in Different Types of Systems

The examples provided in Tables 1.1 and 1.2 do not fully acknowledge the complexity that exists in health and social care systems, but they do provide a framework to start to ensure that the breadth of the system elements is considered. Health and social care systems are dynamic and uncertain settings, generally working with time pressures and a multitude of different staff roles all providing different functions but with the same goal, to enhance patient and client well-being and to ensure safety. This requires embracing the messy reality of what health and social care systems look like, how they must adapt and transcend several clinical and non-clinical settings, and the variability that exists to ensure efficiency and safety are carefully balanced. It requires insight into how different processes may interact, each with their own discrete work systems. This takes our gaze up from the elements at the work system level to interacting work processes.

How closely parts of the system interact and couple together determines how dependent one element of the system is upon another. For example, a nurse may be unable to deliver a drug without a prescription. A poorly completed prescription or drug chart will delay the delivery of the drug. The delivery of a drug and completion of a drug chart can be referred to as 'tightly coupled' – tasks that are dependent upon each other but can be two discrete processes, completed by different members of the team.

Health and social care systems do not all benefit from a clear sequence or dependency between processes or tasks. A patient may arrive in an emergency department, where speed is required to take a blood sample to inform how the patient should be treated. Who takes the samples, completes the request for tests and sends the bloods for testing may vary, depending on how staff are required to support the patient. In another context, where blood may be taken in a GP's practice or by a phlebotomist on a ward, the sequence of tasks and a single member of staff will be consistent through the whole process. Some systems can be described as 'loosely coupled', and this implies a greater level of variability, in terms of their sequence, timing, the person doing the work and even how the work is done. Why does this matter? Understanding the context is important for understanding how the system usually succeeds. Variability in loosely coupled systems can be a positive characteristic, as it allows the system to respond to variable demands or shifts in system priorities. Health and social care systems have to adapt to accommodate the needs of many patients and clients, the time pressure associated with certain conditions or tasks, or the availability of resources within the organisation, such as, for example, specific staff skills or access to organisational services in responding to a deteriorating patient or managing the delivery of a baby.

These two different properties of a system, loose or tight coupling, influence how we focus our improvements (Vincent and Amalberti, 2016). They require different approaches to support patient safety and staff well-being. In tightly coupled systems, the predictability of how tasks are completed can support the use of rules and procedures to reduce the risk of harm. However, even the best procedural intervention can be overused or misused. Organisations will often assume a level of performance and safety based on the library it holds of up-to-date policies and procedures. When we take a closer look and count the number of pages of all the policies and procedures that a single member of staff is required to recall, relevant to their field of work, it becomes quickly apparent that it is highly unlikely that the human brain can remember all these details. Even asking staff to show you where to find all the relevant policies and procedures can present a challenge for them. This makes an excellent activity to try when going into a new work environment: ask staff to locate a selection of policies, and ask their opinion on how practically achievable those policies are at all times of the day or week in all contexts. This may illustrate issues of accessibility or usability in how policies and procedures are stored or written.

Observing how work is really done, we find reasons why policies and procedures when put into practice may contradict one another or require adjustments by staff to reflect the reality of a work context. This may be due to how practical it is to adhere to the policies within a particular environment, to manage the associated time pressures and to retain compassion and care for patients and service users. For example, staff balancing the need to see many patients in a short period of time, such as in an outpatient clinic, with the amount of time spent with each individual patient. Trade-offs are inevitable, as staff aim to achieve the efficiency required by the organisation to meet performance goals, such as, for example, a defined time period between patient referral and consultation. Clinics may be booked with a large number of patients all allocated a ten-minute appointment, with little room to deviate from timings without that having an impact on the efficiency of the clinic. It may take just one piece of information to not be immediately available and the clinic could stall; except that they do not stall, as staff adapt to and accommodate these less than perfect scenarios. Administrative and clinical staff will work to ensure the patient's care is not impeded, and clinicians work hard to provide consultations, perhaps with incomplete information, to enable the patient to proceed to the next investigation or intervention required.

When working in a safety role, spending time in different work environments can help understand why policies and procedures may not always be achievable or are unlikely to be adhered to. This is rarely down to a blatant disregard by staff or to just one factor in the system, but rather results from a combination of how the organisation responds to performance measures, availability of staff, effectiveness of equipment and tools relied upon, physical environments and even the unpredictability of the work and people within the system. So, the question is how many of the policies and procedures are critical to the tasks completed? Some procedures will always be essential for safety-critical and clearly defined tasks, but how else can safety be achieved, and is there a better way other than resorting to writing another procedure?

In the context of a loosely coupled system and situations where unpredictability is high, time pressure likely, and the reliability of information varies, a more dynamic approach to working efficiently and safely is required. This requires an organisation to respond with a greater emphasis placed upon supporting staff to be able to make and execute decisions and tasks in a reasonable way, balancing potentially competing priorities. A proactive approach to recognising local issues and addressing organisational, environmental and equipment challenges can assist in increasing the preparedness and resilience within the system to enable staff to work and make decisions well. How reliable and quick are IT systems in obtaining and prompting staff to information that may support their decision making? Do the physical environment and process of procurement and restocking of equipment assist staff and patients to receive the most appropriate equipment within the required timeframe? Does the organisation or the wider system ensure rostering or access to testing and scanning facilities that enable staff to increase the knowledge used to inform their clinical judgement and intervention? The resources available and the workload created by the demands associated with patient care will influence the scale of trade-offs made by staff or mistaken selections of equipment required, as efficiency is prioritised over quality and accuracy.

The context of a health and social care environment will determine which aspect of the work system is most significant or compromised relative to a particular process. HF/E looks to address how the system influences performance, safety and well-being. The trade-off of time versus efficiency, and of efficiency versus quality, is important to acknowledge to develop realistic and suitable safety and quality improvements, while acknowledging the remaining risks.

Not all risks can be removed – that is the reality of managing performance and safety in dynamic and uncertain systems – but we should aim to have knowledge of the risk and support an approach to manage and reduce it. HF/E can help organisations obtain a transparent log of the risks specific to different work systems, to clarify where the responsibility for that risk lies within the organisation and ensure frontline staff are supported by the organisation through acknowledgement and management of the remaining risks. Health and social care professionals are obviously accountable for their individual competency and skills to optimise service-user and patient safety and to manage risks. Organisations are accountable for the ability of the professional to obtain and deliver these skills in the context of the system. Organisations manage the risk created or inherent to the work system. HF/E can support system design to enable staff, patients and service users to interact safely and efficiently and to optimise the well-being of all.

How Do We Do HF/E?

The simple answer is that there are many different methods and tools used to understand different systems (see, for example, Stanton et al., 2013, for a practical overview of a large number of HF/E methods). The approach to recognising safety issues in technology may look different from understanding how communication influences a task, and different again if we are considering the flow and design of a specific health and social care process or environment. Some methods lend themselves to the collection of quantitative and measurable data, for example considering improvements in the efficiency of a task or the reduction of a specific incident reported or staff injury. However, if we are interested in well-being, workload or fatigue, these factors may rely on qualitative and quantitative evaluation. Methods and tools can be learnt or developed over time, but the priority for health and social care is to understand the principles of the systems approach, which HF/E adopts as a way to look at improving outcomes, such as the safety of service users, patients and staff.

Quality improvement (QI) has become well established as an approach to address patient safety. This has enabled many staff to be effective in addressing workplace challenges. The difference in mindset needs to be appreciated to understand why HF/E may complement existing QI strategies (Hignett et al., 2015). QI has traditionally focused on the efficiency of the system and the adoption of best practice, focusing on the standardisation of normal work practices. HF/E considers a broader range of outcomes, including safety and well-being. These outcomes are addressed through recognising the predictable and unpredictable contexts, specific to an industry's systems, to identify where to focus resources to reduce or mitigate risks and to improve interactions of the different elements of the system.

There are similarities and differences between QI and HF/E approaches (Table 1.3); however, these should not be pitched against each other, as both can benefit health and social care systems.

TABLE 1.3 Characteristics of QI and HF/E

	QI	HF/E
Focus	Process	Safety, well-being, performance
Investigations	Data driven	Observation and analysis of work
Approach	System and participatory	System and participatory
Solutions	Modify process, teams, training	Redesign: tasks, equipment, environment and system

Recognising the strengths of each, and the most appropriate time to apply them, is the most constructive use of the methods familiar to each discipline. Now is the time to optimise both; HF/E has a focus on understanding the complexity of system and what is required to design safety into the system, while QI can support the process and evaluation of change in the system. Drawing an analogy to clinical practice, HF/E offers a diagnostic approach to the hazards, risks and opportunities (pathology), which exist in the system (environment, tasks, equipment, people and organisation), adopting a multi-disciplinary team (staff, patients, all users) approach to design. QI has the tools and instruments to implement changes, and to assess whether the change adopted is effective in achieving the intended outcome. When combining QI and HF/E we should look for outcomes that encompass the aims of both disciplines: seeking to reduce harm through reduced risk, increasing efficiency through enhanced processes, and optimising staff well-being.

A challenge can arise if outcome measures drive the focus of change and are selected based solely on their ability to visually present quantitative change. The messy reality of health and social care systems must be acknowledged, and understanding the problem should ultimately determine the focus of change. Managing performance and safety in any safety-critical industry does not lend itself easily to randomised controlled trials, which are best suited to situations where there are a limited number of variables to control and measure. Improvements in complex systems obviously require evaluation, but outcome measures should be selected based on the perception of value to the patient, staff and organisation and should be intrinsically linked to knowledge in enhancing the performance and safety of complex sociotechnical systems.

An HF/E approach rarely relies on just one piece of information to explore or explain a work context. The triangulation of information from a mix of methods is more likely to ensure a richer insight and focus on how best to evaluate the effectiveness of any subsequent intervention. Equally important is the understanding that all perspectives are relevant. The clinical perspective is significantly valuable but cannot provide the whole picture. Administrative staff, patients porters, cleaners and those who are intermittently present in an environment provide the benefit of understanding how different parts of the system function or how the same task is done differently by different staff members; for example, the routine task of patient identification may be achieved differently, with some staff groups adopting safer strategies, which could be shared and standardised by an organisation. The voice of the patient and relative is equally key, as intentions and perspectives of those delivering a service may not always align with those receiving it; measuring improvement needs to reflect how different users suggest what could be classified as an improvement from their perspective.

The design and development of any intervention should seek to adopt a co-design or participatory approach, engaging all relevant stakeholders. However, HF/E interventions also integrate science and evidence, identified as relevant to the issue. The use of evidence is essential to recognise the strength or likelihood of success for any improvement intervention introduced. Interventions to control risks, for example, can vary in form and strength; matching a risk control intervention to the potential for harm is based on the evidence of effectiveness and available resources. There are a few key principles applicable with any design process, and these include the need to understand the context and users to develop a potential solution, while continuously evaluating and reiterating any design until an acceptable solution is found. HF/E relies on these principles to modify and adapt solutions, rather than expect a solution previously adopted in another area to be immediately effective. One size will not fit all contexts in health and social care.

Chapter Summary

This chapter introduced you to the principles of a systems approach used within HF/E. Table 1.4 summarises key systems-thinking principles. You have been provided with a systems framework, SEIPS, to support this way of thinking. This should enable you to review an area in health and social care and consider which elements of the system interact with each other, and how those interactions make it easier or harder for professionals to work and maintain effective performance and safety. You were introduced to differences in how systems may interact, and where different approaches to improving performance and safety might be required. This chapter has started introducing the idea of blending QI and HF/E together, acknowledging that health and social care systems are messy, which requires a proactive approach to understanding the context of a system and its risks and opportunities to inform how to design improvements. The remainder of the book will provide practical guidance on how to look at each element of the work system illustrated within SEIPS. The only way to fully understand where and how HF/E can support patient safety, performance and well-being is to take a leap of faith and try some of the ideas presented within the book. Everything shared in this book has been used in health and social care settings by the authors, but more importantly the presented approaches are applied widely across industries to understand and improve outcomes.

TABLE 1.4 Summary of systems-thinking principles and how they are addressed within HF/E

Systems-thinking principle	Application within HF/E
The boundary and properties of the system are stated.	Recognise the limits and characteristics of the system to inform the method and resources required to understand interactions and how performance, well-being and safety can be best achieved.
Interactions of system elements will create emergent properties for system performance and safety.	Understanding the nature and impact of system element interactions should inform HF/E analysis to support system design to improve, manage or mitigate factors influencing safety, performance or well-being.
A systems approach reduces blame in the context of an incident.	People are just one part of the system. Understanding which elements are most influential or likely to have contributed to a particular outcome provides context for actions and outcomes. Seek to understand the local rationality and why things made sense at the time.

(continued)

TABLE 1.4 (*continued*)

Systems-thinking principle	Application within HF/E
Health and social care are complex adaptive systems.	Recognising the variability, dependencies and coupling between different parts of the system can inform how best to manage inherent risks and respond to opportunities.
A user-centred design approach is fundamental to improve system performance.	Applying methods and approaches to incorporate a wide group of stakeholders in understanding and developing system change.

CIEHF HF/E Competencies

Use of a human-centred approach to the design and development of systems
- Understands the role and application of HF/E principles in optimising system performance and well-being across all ages and capabilities.

Focus on how other system components and performance-influencing factors affect people
- Understands the theoretical and practice bases for analysis of human interactions.

Human characteristics, capabilities and limitations
- Understands the theoretical and practice bases for HF/E relating to physical capabilities and limitations.

References

Carayon, P., Wooldridge, A., Hoonakker, P., et al. 2020. SEIPS 3.0: Human-centered design of the patient journey for patient safety. *Applied Ergonomics*, 84, 103033.

Donabedian, A. 1988. The quality of care: How can it be assessed? *Journal of the American Medical Association*, 260, 1743–1748.

Hignett, S., Jones, E. L., Miller, D., et al. 2015. Human factors and ergonomics and quality improvement science: Integrating approaches for safety in healthcare. *BMJ Quality & Safety*, 24, 250.

Holden, R. J., Carayon, P., Gurses, A. P., et al. 2013. SEIPS 2.0: A human factors framework for studying and improving the work of healthcare professionals and patients. *Ergonomics*, 56, 1669–1686.

Holden, R. J. & Carayon, P. 2021. SEIPS 101 and seven simple SEIPS tools. *BMJ Quality & Safety*, 30, 901–910.

Russ, A. L., Fairbanks, R. J., Karsh, B.-T., et al. 2013. The science of human factors: Separating fact from fiction. *BMJ Quality & Safety*, 22, 802–808.

Stanton, N., Salmon, P. M., Rafferty, L. A., et al. 2013. *Human factors methods: A practical guide for engineering and design*, Ashgate Publishing Ltd.

Vincent, C. & Amalberti, R. 2016. *Safer healthcare: Strategies for the real world*. Springer.

Wilson, J. R. 2014. Fundamentals of systems ergonomics/human factors. *Applied Ergonomics*, 45, 5–13.

Wilson, J. R. & Corlett, E. N. 1995. *Evaluation of Human Work, Second Edition*, CRC Press.

CHAPTER 2

The Organisation

Chapter Objectives and Learning Outcomes

- To describe, in simple terms, the concept of organisational culture, and specifically how safety culture relates to this.
- To recognise features of good safety culture.
- To define key concepts of proactive risk management.
- To introduce methods for assessing safety culture (and consider their strengths and weaknesses).
- Using a worked example, to introduce a tool for helping you to understand and strengthen safety culture in your own organisation.

Introduction: Understanding and Shaping the Role of Your Organisation in Defining the Work Context

This book has chosen the Systems Engineering Initiative for Patient Safety (SEIPS) as its systems framework. This is described in detail in Chapter 1, but we can summarise it as having two fundamental elements. The first is that outcomes (including efficiency, safety and well-being) are delivered as result of processes. Second, the specific nature of these processes arises from the work context in which they are delivered. The work context is described in SEIPS as the 'work system' elements and the 'interactions' between them. The organisation is just one element, but its contribution to context is particularly strong, because of its influence on the other elements. For example, the organisation will make procurement decisions that affect the tools and technologies available to staff, while staffing will be influenced by workforce planning at an organisational level. Estates and infrastructure planning (and procurement) will directly influence the physical environment in which care is delivered, while organisational attitudes to risk and safety permeate every other aspect of the work system.

Improvement interventions that do not consider the organisational contribution to context are much less likely to be successful, and also limit the potential for wider learning. A good example of this is provided by Dixon-Woods and Martin in their reflection on the impact of Quality Improvement interventions, specifically in relation to the implementation of sepsis bundles (Dixon-Woods and Martin, 2016).

> **BOX 2.1** Elements of the sepsis bundle
>
> 1. Deliver high-flow oxygen.
> 2. Take blood cultures.
> 3. Administer empiric intravenous antibiotics.
> 4. Measure serum lactate and send full blood count.
> 5. Start intravenous fluid resuscitation.
> 6. Commence accurate urine output measurement.

These bundles require organisations to deliver on six clinical activities within the first hour after sepsis is suspected (Box 2.1).

On the surface, these make sense and appear straightforward, but in reality may be anything but, depending on the organisational context. You can see that the need for laboratory testing and antibiotic supply means that your local care delivery system (the ward environment) needs to interact with other systems, such as pharmacy and clinical biochemistry. Access to these (and the effectiveness of your engagement with them) is likely to be affected by factors beyond your immediate control. Within organisations that have delivered successfully on sepsis bundles, it is likely that there are a whole host of 'facilitating conditions', which may well not be present in a different organisation. Reports of interventions that do not acknowledge such contextual factors are not helpful for other organisations. Why don't we routinely report on such factors? Facilitating factors are often invisible – if we approach a well-designed door, the information that tells us how to use it is built in, and we will pass through the door without even really being aware of how we opened and closed it (Norman, 2013). The same is true for organisational facilitators, and if we don't know how to actively identify them, then they often remain hidden.

A second issue is that many of these organisational factors are considerably less tangible than the design features of a door. They emerge from the values, attitudes and deep-seated practices across all levels of the organisation. They are part of what it is often described as 'culture'. This is one of the more challenging areas when you are new to HF/E. Even experienced specialists struggle to define and understand culture. Catchpole (2014) observes that 'the idea of culture is perhaps similar to the idea of "intelligence" – everyone thinks they know what it is, but conceptual clarity is more elusive', while Reason (1997) is perhaps somewhat more blunt in saying that it has 'the definitional precision of a cloud'.

The aim of this chapter is to help you consider aspects of organisational culture and development that are likely to impact on performance and, particularly, on safety, as well as to introduce tools that may be useful for you in assessing safety culture within your own organisation. Given that organisational factors strongly shape context, they are often considered 'performance-influencing factors', and examples include staffing, workload and fatigue management, as can be seen in the delivery of the NHS Health Check, introduced in Box 2.2 and discussed later in the chapter.

Chapter 2　The Organisation

BOX 2.2　Example – the NHS Health Check – organisational influences

> Despite relative success across the UK in achieving a reduction in morbidity and mortality relating to cardiovascular disease, it is still a major killer, claiming the lives of over 124,000 people in England during 2017. The NHS Health Check, introduced in 2009, is the largest preventative intervention for cardiovascular disease in the UK, and is based on the theory that identifying high-risk individuals and optimising primary care prevention has a knock-on effect on reducing population risk. There is a quantitative relationship between risk factors and disease incidence. High-quality longitudinal research studies have allowed this relationship to be mathematically modelled, underpinning cardiovascular 'risk engines', which measure individual risk and how it changes following intervention. The NHS Health Check is offered to all people in England between the ages of 40 and 74 years, and it involves taking a detailed client history and some simple point-of-care testing, including measurement of blood pressure, body mass index, blood lipid levels (specifically total- and high-density-lipoprotein (HDL)-cholesterol), as well as blood glucose. These data are entered into the risk engine, which returns an estimate of the ten-year risk of a cardiovascular event, such as stroke or heart attack. The aim of the service is risk stratification: identifying those with existing disease – or at a high risk of developing it – and referring them for treatment, while those at low to moderate risk are encouraged to make diet and lifestyle changes to reduce or maintain their risk status, returning every five years for further assessment.
>
> The outcomes are not strong, given the high programme costs (Kypridemos et al., 2018); only small decreases in modelled risk are achieved, and it has been estimated that this translates into the prevention of one clinical event for every 4,762 attendees. To look at it another way, this means the prevention of 1,400 events across the whole country for each five-year cycle.
>
> It is worthy of note that there was some scepticism surrounding the inception of the programme – it was felt that the evidence base supporting the population benefits of targeting individual risk was not strong (Martin et al., 2018). Has this misgiving been borne out in practice, or are there other factors at play? It is recognised that there are wide variations in service delivery, which are at least in part due to differences in local implementation, influenced by organisational factors. The use of safety culture discussion cards (described later) allows the unpacking of barriers and facilitators to cardiovascular risk management.

Consideration of the organisational context should be the starting point for any activity, but this approach might also be of particular use for:

- Patient safety incident responses
- Designing new procedures
- Procurement
- Initiating a new service
- Reviewing/cessation of a service.

Organisational Culture and Safety Culture

In the large complex organisations that deliver health and social care, organisational culture is not uniform, and is made up of many interwoven subcultures (Mannion and Smith, 2018). Often these are forged along the lines of occupational subgroups, as illustrated by the Morecambe Bay investigation (Kirkup, 2015), or in terms of organisational outcomes, such as safety. These subcultures are impossible to separate – and will share many of the same elements. However, for this chapter we will use the term 'culture' to refer to safety culture in particular.

The birth of the term 'safety culture' is associated with the investigation into the Chernobyl disaster of 1986, although coining the term probably reflected a growing awareness that safety 'belongs to the system' and that major adverse events have both a history and a context that is organisational in nature. If this seems complicated and bit vague, then you would be right – it is – and there are no easy answers to measuring, assessing and improving culture. Over the past century, we have seen a shift in safety thinking (Dekker, 2019), moving from behaviourist scientific management approaches that sought to improve safety and performance by standardising processes and removing variation, to a systems approach (Figure 2.1). The latter recognises that safety is an emergent organisational outcome that depends on so much more than individual attitudes and behaviours; rather, it encompasses the shared thinking, as well as the administrative structures and allocated resources, that embed ideas about what it means to be safe and how an organisation can have confidence that it is operating safely.

Defining what we mean by safety culture is one of the first challenges: this has been the subject of numerous debates, articles and books over the years, but this is beyond the scope of this chapter. However, if the concept of culture is to be useful, it is important to have some understanding of it, and how it relates to the specific work setting under consideration. In the introduction we addressed the concept of emergence – culture is in many ways an emergent outcome of the system that describes the organisation as a whole. Specifically, it emerges from the beliefs, goals and activities of the people within the organisation and across all levels of the organisation. From a practical perspective, Phipps and Ashcroft (2014, p. 100) offer a useful insight that 'at the heart of safety culture is a reciprocal relationship between the effort organisational members put into safety practice and the contentment with what is achieved through these efforts'. Strong safety cultures will, therefore, have structures that support 'double-loop learning'; safety goals will be actively set and performance against these goals assessed regularly. The 'double loop' aspect comes from a continual process of assessment of the goals themselves: are they the right goals for this organisation at the current time?

A small amount of theory is useful in considering the challenges of exploring and changing culture. The references section of this chapter provides links to further reading (such as Dekker, 2012; Guldenmund, 2000; Waterson, 2014), but it is fair to say that most of the models in the literature reflect the concept of culture having multiple layers, often described as an 'onion'. The core of this onion is deeply

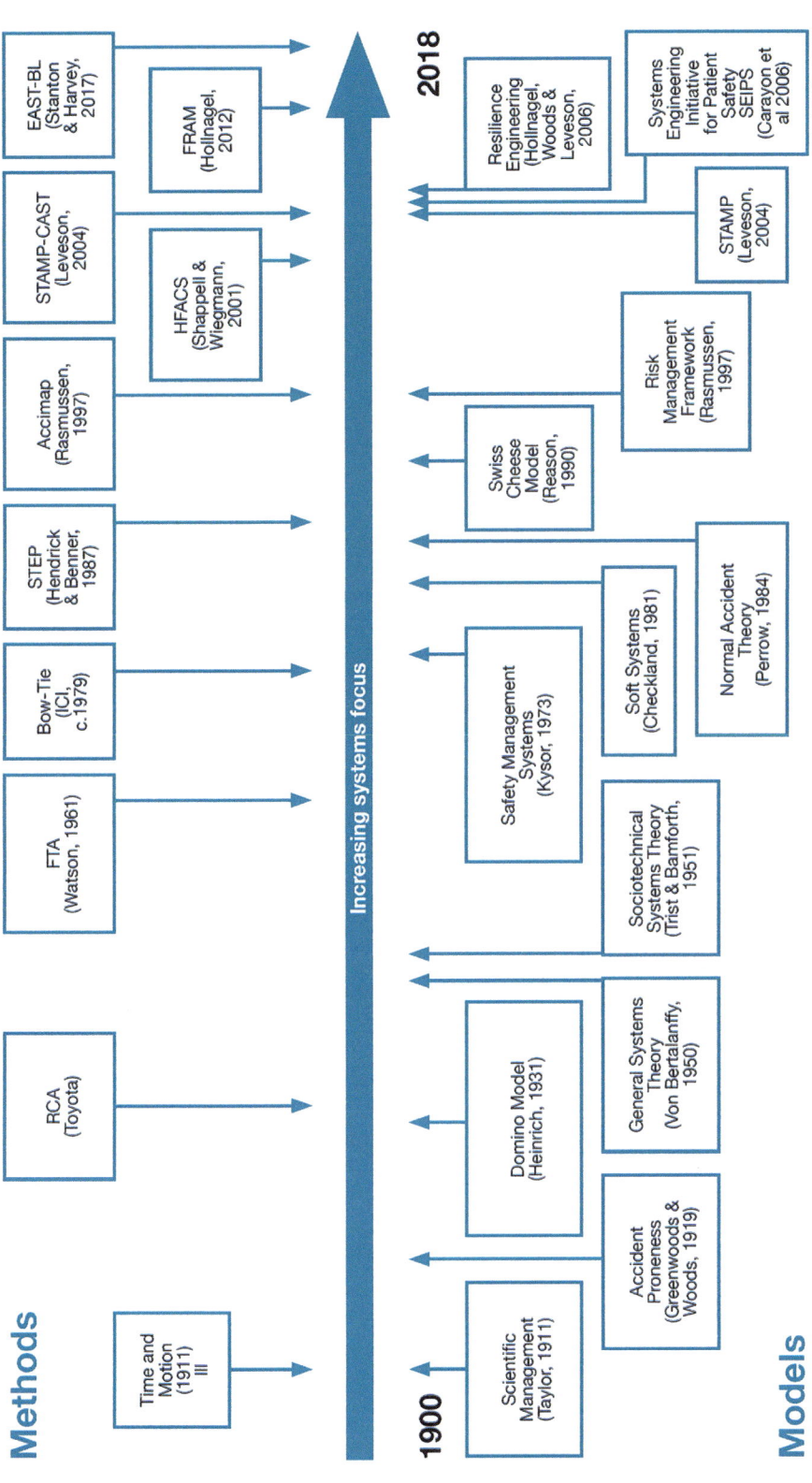

FIGURE 2.1 Timeline showing the evolution of safety thinking towards increasing systems focus.

Source: Adapted from Stanton et al. 2019.

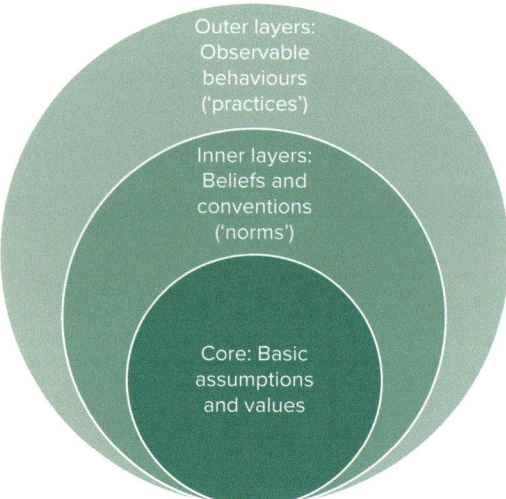

FIGURE 2.2 Summary of the core principle of current culture models.

hidden, and this presents challenges both in terms of understanding and describing it, but also in terms of changing it. The deepest layer is fundamental, even pre-conscious, and members of the group may not even articulate these assumptions and values and may not even recognise why they are so important to them. 'Norms' are the agreed expectations that guide the behaviour of the group, while practices' are the observable behaviours and accessible artefacts, such as policies and procedures. Exploring and influencing the outer layer will ultimately influence the core. However, the core strongly influences the outer layers, which are easier to observe. While the relationship between the layers is not straightforward to understand, the literature also contains well-made arguments that indicate starting with the outer layers – usually considered to be the 'observable practices' of the organisation (Figure 2.2) – is the only way to bring about change within a reasonable timeframe.

Another aspect of theory that might be useful in thinking about 'practical culture' is recognising that culture development is an evolutionary survival mechanism – for groups of people to have a shared understanding (albeit completely implicit) means that any individual knows how people in this group are expected to behave. They, therefore, know how they should themselves behave – it is part of an adaptation to environmental change. Understanding the history of your organisation and the pressures that have shaped it can give you an insight into culture. It follows from the notion that 'culture reflects history' that culture is also a form of organisational memory, indicating that culture is 'learnt'. This is important to be aware of – new people coming into the organisation will not have been directly affected by previous change, but they will learn their responses based on what they observe in the workplace, which might not necessarily be appropriate or desirable. A final point worth considering is that culture within an organisation is not likely to be homogenous. Culture belongs to groups, and organisations are made up of individuals who are part of other groups, and each of these groups will have

Chapter 2   The Organisation

BOX 2.3   Example – cultural layers exposed during the Morecambe Bay Investigation into maternity services

> 'Morecambe Bay' was an investigation into the management, delivery and outcomes of care provided by the maternity and neonatal services at the University Hospitals of Morecambe Bay NHS Foundation Trust from June 2004 to June 2013. The investigation was led by Dr Bill Kirkup CBE (Kirkup, 2015). In terms of outcomes, there were 20 instances of what were considered 'significant or major failures of care' at Furness General Hospital, and these were associated with three maternal deaths and the death of 16 babies. It was considered that different clinical care could have prevented twelve of these deaths (one mother and eleven babies). The investigation considered culture to be a significant factor, and although this was complex and difficult to unpick, there were some specific aspects that are useful in illustrating the layers described in Figure 2.2. The investigation began with *tangible artefacts*, including incident investigation reports. These revealed poor practice: for example, almost all investigations were carried out by the same senior midwife, and they were almost invariably uni-disciplinary in nature; there was evidence of blame-shifting behaviour that aimed to protect the midwifery team; and there was little evidence of dissemination of these findings to support organisational learning. Risk assessment practices also appeared inadequate in identifying babies and mothers at higher risk. Further investigation uncovered an *apparent norm* within the midwifery team that could be described as 'keep obstetricians away'; obstetricians were often not informed that a mother was delivering, and they were not contacted even when it became apparent that complications were unfolding. This may seem difficult to understand, but at the heart of this behaviour was a deep belief that birth had become over-medicalised and this impacted negatively on both mothers and babies. Many people would empathise with this perspective, but it appears that the relevant *shared value* of the midwifery team had become 'normal birth at all cost'. This is a problem, because while birth is undoubtedly a normal physiological process, it is also inherently risky with a relatively high frequency of life-threatening complications, and medical intervention does save lives.

their own values, norms and practices. Culture clashes may contribute to adverse events, as illustrated by the poor relationships between midwives and obstetricians described in Box 2.3.

What Does a Positive Safety Culture Look Like?

Safety culture is often described as multi-dimensional, and there is acceptance that any organisation culture is unlikely to be equally developed in every dimension. This has led to the development of assessment tools that define dimensions and require organisations to 'score' themselves in respect of these dimensions (Table 2.1). There is not necessarily any agreed position on what constitutes a positive safety culture, so the dimensions on which each of these tools are based differ. However,

TABLE 2.1 Frequently used safety culture/climate assessment tools

Tool	Type	Dimensions	Notes
Safety Attitudes Questionnaire (SAQ) (Sexton et al., 2006)	Quantitative	Teamwork climate Job satisfaction Perceptions of management Safety climate Working conditions Stress recognition	The majority of the questionnaire consists of Likert-scaled responses. However, there is also a free-text response question: 'What are your top three recommendations for improving patient safety in this clinical area?'
Safety, Communication, Operational Reliability and Engagement (SCORE) (Sexton et al., 2019)	Quantitative	Improvement readiness Local leadership Burnout climate and personal burnout Teamwork climate Safety climate	This tool is a development of the SAQ and has a broader focus. There are additional sections that explore growth opportunities, workload, participation in decision making, job-related uncertainty and career advancement.
Safety Culture Index (Spurgeon et al., 2019)	Quantitative	Coping with work demands Participation in decision making Checking and accountability Commitment to learning Purpose and direction Working in collaboration Sharing information Blame-free climate Role clarity Staff motivation Standards monitoring Vision and mission	Dimensions are divided as belonging to the individual, to the team and to the organisation. This division recognises that organisations are hierarchical, and so culture can be assessed at multiple levels. The matrix also recognises four different working contexts: **Task** focus, **people** focus, **controls** focus and **change** focus.
Patient Safety Culture in Healthcare Organisations (Singer et al., 2007)	Quantitative	Senior manager engagement Organisational resources Overall emphasis on safety Unit safety norms	Dimensions are divided as belonging to the organisation, to units within the organisation, and to the individual. Together, they produce the ninth dimension of the 'provision of safe care'.

Chapter 2 The Organisation

Tool	Type	Dimensions	Notes
		Unit recognition and support for safety	
		Fear of shame	
		Fear of blame	
		Learning	
Hospital Survey on Patient Safety Culture (Sorra and Nieva, 2004)	Quantitative	Teamwork across hospital units	In addition to the Likert-scaled responses, participants are asked to award an overall grade on patient safety for their work area/unit and to indicate the number of reported events in the past year.
		Teamwork within units	
		Hospital handoffs and transitions	
		Frequency of event reporting	
		Non-punitive response to error	
		Communication openness	
		Feedback and communication about error	
		Organisational learning and continuous improvement	
		Supervisor/manager expectations and actions promoting patient safety	
		Hospital management support for patient safety	
		Staffing	
		General perceptions of safety	
Safety Climate Survey (Sexton et al., 2000)	Quantitative	Senior managers' engagement	This is a questionnaire developed for aviation and applied in healthcare.
		Organisational resources for safety	
		Overall emphasis on safety	
		Unit manager support	
		Unit safety norms	
		Unit recognition for support and safety efforts	
		Collective learning	

(continued)

TABLE 2.1 (*continued*)

Tool	Type	Dimensions	Notes
		Problem responsiveness Fear of blame and punishment Provision of safe care	
GP-SafeQuest (de Wet et al., 2010)	Quantitative	Workload Communication Leadership Teamwork Safety systems	As many of the other instruments recognise, the term 'organisational culture' subsumes multiple subcultures. This tool was devised to support understanding of team culture in primary care settings.
Manchester Patient Safety Assessment Framework (MaPSaF) (Kirk et al., 2007)	Qualitative	Commitment to overall continuous improvement Priority given to safety System errors and individual responsibility Recording incidents and best practice Evaluating incidents and best practice Learning and effecting change Communication about safety issues Personnel management and safety issues Staff education and training Team working	The tool has been adapted for a number of different care settings. It is widely used across England and Wales. It encourages discussion and assessment of safety culture maturity.
Safety Culture Discussion Cards (NHS Education for Scotland (NES), 2024)	Exploratory	Leadership and management commitment Resourcing Just culture, reporting and learning Risk awareness and management Teamwork Communication Responsibility Involvement	The cards move away from measurement and support the wider discussion that facilitates deeper understanding of safety as an emergent outcome of a health and care system.

Chapter 2 The Organisation

there is considerable overlap, and dimensions that are contained within many tools include:

- Leadership commitment to safety (at all levels of leadership from board level through to managers and supervisors working with frontline staff)
- A shared belief in the importance of safety across all levels of the organisation
- Open communication founded on trust
- Open reporting systems, where staff are comfortable about reporting adverse events without fear of punishment
- Commitment to organisational learning (including learning from near misses and normal work as well as from adverse events)
- A strong strategic approach to risk and safety management
- Good teamwork and inter-professional team working
- Conditions that support safe working
- Adequate staffing (and other resourcing)
- Understanding the importance of staff well-being
- Recognition of stress/burnout
- Understanding fatigue
- Quality of handovers.

Measuring Performance

It follows from what has been discussed previously that the safety culture dimensions of an organisation are likely to describe its more superficial cultural layers. Most of the tools outlined in Table 2.1 are designed as questionnaires, usually gauging opinion through use of Likert scales. These data are treated numerically, with mean scores being calculated for each of the items in the questionnaire (hence the use of the term 'quantitative' in Table 2.1). The questionnaires are usually restricted to no more than two sides of A4 to avoid making them too onerous. The short timeframe for answering means that results are very much a snapshot of these surface features, and this is what is meant by 'safety climate', although the term is often used interchangeably with culture.

However, quantitative measurement is not the only approach available to consider safety culture. Semi-quantitative approaches have been used in the NHS, and, more recently, qualitative exploration of safety culture has become increasingly popular. The Manchester Patient Safety Assessment Framework (MaPSaF) (Kirk et al., 2007) is an example of a semi-quantitative approach. It is designed to support discussions about safety culture among teams, with a view to organisations using the results to position themselves along a maturity axis from pathological to generative as described in Table 2.2. The greater degree of engagement in this approach is likely to involve a deeper dive into safety culture, and if the results of the discussions are formally captured and analysed, this will give some insight into starting points for improvements. It is worthy of note that the dimensions themselves may need further unpacking if staff are to fully understand them. This is done within all the tools – for the questionnaires, each dimension has several items within it that clarify what is being asked. The MaPSaF handbook contains prompts for each dimension to support further understanding and discussion. However – especially for the questionnaires – individual interpretation may affect the results.

TABLE 2.2 Safety culture maturity axis (based on Westrum, 1993)

Maturity state	Characteristics
Pathological	Staff at all levels care less about safety than the need to be seen to comply with regulatory requirements and not be caught out in terms of infringements. Staff are actively discouraged from highlighting safety issues and reporting incidents. Where reporting happens, it is flawed, limited in scope and there is little or no wider dissemination to support organisational learning.
Reactive	Safety activity is driven almost entirely in response to incidents.
Bureaucratic	The organisation has implemented a structured risk management system, but it tends to be a 'box-ticking' exercise, and the results used as evidence to demonstrate the safety of the system. Rather than engaging the whole workforce, safety efforts are seen as belonging to an individual safety manager or team.
Proactive	The organisation actively seeks out safety information to support the development of its safety management system, and the use of this information is explicit and transparent.
Generative	Safety is embedded across the organisation, and everyone understands their role in improvement. Key to improvement is honesty about failure, and this is supported by a non-punitive reporting system.

All the tools have limitations: they largely represent 'expert opinion' rather than demonstrating a clear link to an underpinning theory, and elements have been transposed from other sectors without clear evidence to indicate that this is justified. The strength of the related psychometric properties (content, criterion and construct validity, as well as reliability) is variable. Choice should depend on your intended purpose and your target population, as well as the reported psychometric properties, but the results can be supported using tools like the Safety Culture Discussion Cards described later in this chapter. The more commonly used tools have been listed in Table 2.1.

Ultimately, any safety culture assessment will only be of value if it can be linked directly to outcomes, and very few studies of safety culture seek to do this. However, in recent years, some studies have indicated a link between a positive safety culture and better patient outcomes. Perhaps even more encouraging are recent observations that *changing* culture can improve outcomes, as shown in the 'Leadership saves lives' study, where cultural change was associated with significant decreases in risk-standardised mortality in relation to myocardial infarction (Braithwaite et al., 2017; Mannion and Davies, 2018).

Chapter 2 The Organisation

Health and Social Care Safety Culture Discussion Cards

If you choose a quantitative method for assessing your safety culture, you will be left with a series of scores, which need to be unpacked if they are to be useful for directing improvement. Even the semi-quantitative approach underpinning MaPSaF is limited (as all the tools are) in that it is a snapshot in time. You can augment your safety culture assessment by keeping discussions about safety alive across all levels of your organisation, and a practical way of doing that is through use of the *Health and Social Care Safety Culture Discussion Cards* (NHS Education for Scotland (NES), 2024) developed by NHS Education for Scotland, based on cards developed previously by EUROCONTROL (an intergovernmental organisation for air traffic management across Europe). The cards are arranged under eight dimensions (Box 2.4).

The pack includes guidance and suggestions for how the cards might be used, but suggested approaches are shown in Table 2.3. The easiest way ('safety moments') is to include regular safety culture discussions in team meetings. At each meeting, a new card can be chosen for discussion and reflection, allowing for focused and ongoing dialogue about safety practices.

BOX 2.4 Dimensions covered in the Safety Culture Discussion Cards

	Dimension
	Leadership and management commitment: for example, commitment, priorities and trust.
	Resourcing: for example, getting help, upskilling and training for change.
	Just culture, reporting and learning: for example, speaking up, following the trend and learning from incidents.
	Risk awareness and management: for example, safe procedures, knowing one's risks and balancing safety.
	Teamwork: for example, working together, consulting and talking about systems.
	Communication: for example, sharing, looking outside and breaking down barriers.
	Responsibility: for example, knowing one's relevance to safety, taking responsibility and colleague commitment.
	Involvement: for example, getting involved, making a difference and contributing to change and improvement.

TABLE 2.3 Suggested ways of using the Safety Culture cards ... but feel free to improvise!

Option for use	Details of approach
Comparing views	Different members of your team can sort cards into two piles: what we do well and what we need to improve (your 'team' may be your organisation unit, professional group, etc.). Then compare the piles and discuss: • Where do we agree? • Where do we disagree? • What are the priority issues to address? • What might happen if they are not addressed? • How can this be done? • Who needs to be involved (responsible, consulted, informed)? • When does it need to be done?
Safety moments	In a small group, take just one card – any card. Discuss the card for a set time, such as 15–30 minutes. Discuss a different card each time. Alternatively, in a longer session, allow each person to choose one card from a small selection (for example, from three cards), and ask them to describe an experience that they have had concerning the issue on the card. What can be learnt from their story?
Focus on ...	Choose a specific element, such as 'Resourcing', and discuss each card in depth with your colleagues. You may sort the cards or consider questions such as: • What do we do well? • What and where is our 'best practice' on this issue? • Where have we improved? • Where do we need to improve? • What are we avoiding? • What is stopping us from improving? • How can we improve the situation?
SWOT analysis	Divide the cards into the following piles: • Strengths • Weaknesses • Opportunities • Threats The cards in each pile will tell you something about how safety culture can be improved, by drawing on current strengths, addressing current weaknesses, anticipating and tackling future threats.
Influences	Organise cards into patterns to show how the issues relate to one another. For instance, some cards may have cause-and-effect relationships, or may influence each other in a more subtle way. Discuss how these relationships work.

Chapter 2   The Organisation

In Box 2.2 we introduced the NHS Health Check, a cardiovascular risk management programme, indicating that the outcomes were not strong, with estimates suggesting prevention of relatively few cardiovascular events. Review of the service (generally offered through multiple primary care mechanisms, including via general practice and community pharmacy) suggests that there is significant variation in local implementation, and this may be a factor in limiting effectiveness. An ergonomics study was undertaken to explore community pharmacy delivery of the Health Check, and data were collected using several methods including direct observation, interviews and focus groups (Vosper et al., 2018). As a final phase of the study, the Safety Culture Discussion Cards were used to explore organisational factors with the different teams, using the 'influences' approach. Similar themes were repeated across the different groups and Figure 2.3 shows an example of a related group that was considered particularly important in identifying areas for improving the safety of the Health Check.

Performance-Influencing Factors Relating to Organisational Culture

In Chapter 3 we will introduce the concept of Performance-Influencing Factors (PIFs) as a simple way of considering systems interactions when analysing tasks. Many of these PIFs are related to organisational culture. The safety culture maturity axis is simply describing the behaviours that are 'forced' by the nature of the prevailing culture. For example, while there will be multiple factors contributing to an individual practitioner's fatigue, much of it may arise as a result of organisational factors relating to staff recruitment and retention, which leads to demanding shift patterns. In SEIPS terms, this could be viewed as an external environmental factor – recruitment and retention are recognised as being sector-wide issues. However, how these external issues play out internally will depend on other factors, many of which could be considered organisational. This concept is illustrated in a study into safety culture within community pharmacies (Phipps and Ashcroft, 2014). The study gathered data using a cross-sectional survey of registered community pharmacists in Great Britain. 'Pharmacies' ranged from single independent organisations, right up to large multiples, and the 'pharmacists' spanned the range from locums up to proprietors and branch managers. The survey was a composite of measures related to pharmacist perception of their employment, including effort, reward, job demands, resources available (including support from colleagues and supervisors) and organisational learning. Free-form boxes were also included to capture a qualitative element. Cluster analysis was carried out on the quantitative data. The qualitative data were compared across clusters, allowing the identification of themes common to each cluster, as well as those that 'defined' each cluster. The four clusters identified are shown in Table 2.4.

Much of the data suggested that work demands were related to understaffing, which was viewed both as an external factor and as an organisational factor. This is not surprising, but the identification of the 'challenging pharmacy' is perhaps more so. In this cluster, the work demands are perceived to be particularly high, but this does not appear to have the negative perceived impact on other aspects of the work. Instead,

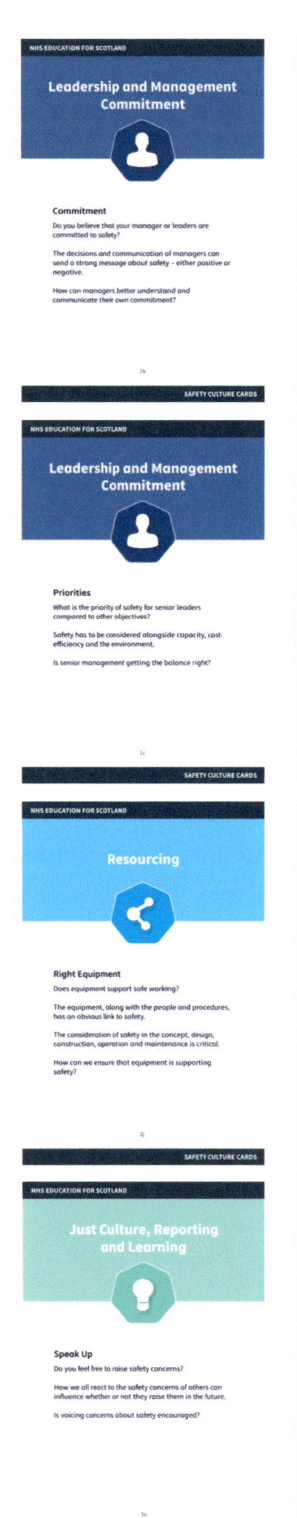

Staff delivering the Health Checks felt that managers didn't really believe in the value of them. This reflected national concerns about the evidence base regarding how individual risk reduction translates into reduced population incidence of cardiovascular events. One participant said that their manager had made the comment 'Well, I'll have retired before the 10 years is up anyway!' Staff felt that these attitudes were reflected in the resourcing that was allocated (see 'Priorities'). While there was some sympathy with this attitude, others pointed out that it would be difficult to build an evidence base if the checks were not carried out to the highest possible standard.

This card brought up several issues which were felt to relate to lack of commitment to the service – for example, in some organisations, it was difficult to ensure that dedicated equipment was available. Often equipment would go missing, only to find it was being used for other activities, sending the message that the Health Check was not important. An important finding arising from this discussion was the limited time allocated for the Check – this turned out to be more than an organisational factor (and may be the driver behind many of the issues): the pharmacist remuneration model still pays pharmacists primarily for dispensing. If the Check took longer than 30 minutes in total, the pharmacy did not make any money.

From the previous card, it seems the risks could be reduced by paying pharmacists properly for providing these services. That is unlikely to happen in the immediate future, so it makes sense to consider other improvements that support safety. The risk engine used for the Health Check requires two blood lipid measurements (total and HDL-cholesterol). Some pharmacies used equipment that required two separate blood samples, each of which took a few minutes to complete, increasing the time pressure. There are machines available (and of suitable accuracy) that allow both readings to be taken from a single sample. This provided a good argument to support future procurement decisions.

The time restriction and the need to take two blood samples (alongside everything else) meant that sometimes bits of the Health Check were missed out. Sometimes this included not measuring HDL-cholesterol. This is potentially dangerous – the Total: HDL-cholesterol ratio is one of the most important predictors of risk. Some staff felt unable to speak up about it as it appeared to be accepted practice. Discussions suggested that the cards had helped them with this – they now had a better understanding of what was driving the behaviour and felt happier to talk about it, as recognising the external pressure made the challenge less confrontational, and they also now had a possible solution.

FIGURE 2.3 Using the Safety Culture Discussion Cards in 'influences' mode.
Source: NHS Education for Scotland (NES), 2024.

Chapter 2 The Organisation

TABLE 2.4 Prototypical safety cultures in pharmacy settings (based on Phipps and Ashcroft, 2014)

Cluster	Defining safety culture characteristics
The disenfranchising pharmacy	Staff feel disengaged from management and perceive that they have little influence on how the pharmacy operates and how services are provided.
The perilous pharmacy	Least favourable scores across the board. High effort and job demands, which are not met by appropriate resourcing. Little sense of personal agency. The organisations most likely to foster patient safety incidents (and the least likely to show evidence of organisational learning).
The safety-focused pharmacy	The most favourable scores across the board, including perception that staff are adequately resourced and supported.
The challenging pharmacy	Generally favourable scores across most aspects of the survey, except for those relating to job demands, which were high compared to the other clusters. However, safety performance was perceived to be good, and staff reported having space and scope to adapt their work to meet demands.

it seems that (whether this is formally agreed or not) people have the space to adapt the work they do to meet demands and deliver acceptable outcomes from the service delivery perspective. The 'acceptance' of adaptation is in itself an organisational resource, but it can be appreciated that it brings with it its own set of risks.

Organisational Resilience

The term 'resilience' is often regarded as an expression of the capability of an individual to manage demands and cope with stress. However, in this book we understand resilience not in terms of the individual but as a set of abilities at the organisational level. The growing field of 'resilient health care' (Hollnagel et al., 2019) builds on work in 'resilience engineering', where resilience is defined as the ability to succeed under varying conditions, with a focus on how organisations cope with complexity and uncertainty in dynamic environments (Woods and Hollnagel, 2006). In healthcare, this has also been interpreted as the ability to adapt to challenges and changes across different levels of a system in order to maintain high-quality care (Wiig et al., 2020).

Adaptations and, more broadly, performance variability are regarded both as inevitable and useful rather than as something that is undesirable. This is because work as described in procedures, standards and protocols is always an abstract, or idealised, representation of how people should carry out their activities, also referred to as work-as-imagined (that is, imagined by those who develop the procedures, standards and protocols). In practice, however, there will always be competing demands and conflicting priorities, uncertainties and ambiguities, which require people to make dynamic trade-offs and judgements (that is, work-as-done) (Sujan et al., 2015). In this respect, there will always be a gap between work-as-imagined and work-as-done (Hollnagel, 2015). It is important that at an organisational level, there is an appreciation of the need for performance variability, as well as processes in place to understand the gap between work-as-imagined and work-as-done.

We can anticipate that having rigid procedures that constrain the ability to adapt are a problem: either adaptation is prevented, or the 'failure to follow procedure' is used against the staff member in a subsequent investigation into an adverse event. This is likely to make people fearful about disclosing adaptations, driving these 'underground' and preventing organisational learning (Debono and Braithwaite, 2015). A better approach is to accept that adaptation keeps complex health and social care systems functioning and to spend time and effort in strengthening resilience abilities. This is firmly within the remit of the organisation.

However, organisational resilience is not just about accepting adaptation — it is about putting processes in place that formally support the development of resilience abilities across all levels of the organisation. Hollnagel defined four key resilience abilities as the ability to (1) monitor, (2) respond, (3) anticipate longer-term changes, treats and opportunities, and (4) learn (Hollnagel, 2010). The safety culture discussion cards are a useful tool in supporting discussions about organisational resilience across all levels of an organisation. In addition, Chapter 9 on Organisational Learning discusses in greater depth the fourth of the resilience abilities and places it into current policy developments in the NHS in England.

Just Culture

Closely related to safety culture is the notion of just culture. The just culture approach aims to strike a balance between not blaming individuals for mistakes and holding them to account for reckless behaviour. Just culture as an organisational response to incidents needs to be underpinned by systems thinking, because the evidence in the literature demonstrates that improvement interventions aimed at the individual are weaker and less effective than systems-based interventions (Kellogg et al., 2017).

Key to applying the principles of just culture is an appropriate understanding of the complexities of everyday work, that is, work-as-done. The notion of accountability, from a systems perspective, is not as much about who is responsible and should be blamed, but rather who can give an account (i.e., provide insight) into what happened and how work is normally carried out. Incident investigation should not be about judgement, but about trying to understand the context, what it was about the environment that made it seem reasonable to those involved to undertake the course of action they selected. If it made sense to this individual, then it is likely to make sense to others working under similar conditions. It is hoped that you can appreciate that many of these actions that come into focus during incident investigation are simply adaptations made by staff trying to deliver successful outcomes in the face of capability–demand mismatches. Human factors and ergonomics approaches seek to uncover this local rationality by trying to understand the conditions within which people work.

Chapter 2 The Organisation

Chapter Summary

People work for and within organisations, and so the culture of those organisations powerfully influences work performance. The ability of the workforce to deliver successful outcomes depends on the work context, and much of that context is defined by the organisational values and the way in which they are reflected in norms and behaviours. Taking time to explore and understand your own organisation allows for a deeper understanding of the barriers to and facilitators of improved performance, safety and well-being.

CIEHF HF/E Competencies

Use of a human-centred approach to the design and development of systems
- Understands the role and application of HF/E principles in optimising system performance and well-being across all ages and capabilities.

Focus on how other system components and performance-influencing factors affect people
- Demonstrates a knowledge of systems theory, including sociotechnical systems and culture (for example, organisational and safety culture).

References

Braithwaite, J., Herkes, J., Ludlow, K., et al. 2017. Association between organisational and workplace cultures, and patient outcomes: Systematic review. *BMJ Open*, 7, e017708.

Catchpole, K. C. 2014. Foreword. In: Waterson, P. (ed.), *Patient safety culture: Theory, methods and application*. Ashgate.

de Wet, C., Spence, W., Mash, R., et al. 2010. The development and psychometric evaluation of a safety climate measure for primary care. *Quality and Safety in Health Care*, 19, 578.

Debono, D. & Braithwaite, J. 2015. Workarounds in nursing practice in acute care: A case of a health care arms race? In: Wears, R., Hollnagel, E. & Braithwaite, J. (eds.), *The resilience of everyday clinical work*. Ashgate.

Dekker, S. 2012. *Just culture: Balancing safety and accountability*. Ashgate.

Dekker, S. 2019. *Foundations of safety science: A century of understanding accidents and disasters*. Routledge.

Dixon-Woods, M. & Martin, G. P. 2016. Does quality improvement improve quality? *Future Hospital Journal*, 3, 191–194.

Guldenmund, F. W. 2000. The nature of safety culture: A review of theory and research. *Safety Science*, 34, 215–257.

Hollnagel, E. 2010. Prologue: The scope of resilience engineering. In: Hollnagel, E., Paries, J., Woods, D. D., et al. (eds.), *Resilience engineering in practice: A guidebook*. Ashgate.

Hollnagel, E. 2015. Why is work-as-imagined different from work-as-done? In: Wears, R., Hollnagel, E. & Braithwaite, J. (eds.), *The resilience of everyday clinical work*. Ashgate.

Hollnagel, E., Sujan, M. & Braithwaite, J. 2019. Resilient health care – Making steady progress. *Safety Science*, 120, 781–782.

Kellogg, K. M., Hettinger, Z., Shah, M., et al. 2017. Our current approach to root cause analysis: Is it contributing to our failure to improve patient safety? *BMJ Quality & Safety*, 26, 381–387.

Kirk, S., Parker, D., Claridge, T., et al. 2007. Patient safety culture in primary care: Developing a theoretical framework for practical use. *Quality and Safety in Health Care*, 16, 313.

Kirkup, B. 2015. *The report of the Morecambe Bay Investigation*. The Morecambe Bay Investigation.

Kypridemos, C., Collins, B., McHale, P., et al. 2018. Future cost-effectiveness and equity of the NHS Health Check cardiovascular disease prevention programme: Microsimulation modelling using data from Liverpool, UK. *PLOS Medicine*, 15, e1002573.

Mannion, R. & Davies, H. 2018. Understanding organisational culture for healthcare quality improvement. *British Medical Journal*, 363, k4907.

Mannion, R. & Smith, J. 2018. Hospital culture and clinical performance: Where next? *BMJ Quality & Safety*, 27, 179.

Martin, A., Saunders, C. L., Harte, E., et al. 2018. Delivery and impact of the NHS Health Check in the first 8 years: A systematic review. *British Journal of General Practice*, 68, e449.

NHS Education for Scotland (NES). 2024. *Safety Culture Discussion Cards*. https://learn.nes.nhs.scot/79396

Norman, D. 2013. *The design of everyday things: Revised and expanded edition*. MIT Press.

Phipps, D. L. & Ashcroft, D. M. 2014. Looking behind patient safety culture: Organisational dynamics, job characteristics and the work domain. In: Waterson, P. (ed.), *Patient safety culture: Theory, methods and application*. CRC Press.

Reason, J. 1997. *Managing the risks of organizational accidents*. Ashgate.

Sexton, J. B., Thomas, E. J. & Helmreich, R. L. 2000. Error, stress, and teamwork in medicine and aviation: Cross sectional surveys. *British Medical Journal*, 320, 745.

Sexton, J. B., Helmreich, R. L., Neilands, T. B., et al. 2006. The Safety Attitudes Questionnaire: Psychometric properties, benchmarking data, and emerging research. *BMC Health Services Research*, 6, 44.

Sexton, J. B., Frankel, A., Leonard, M., et al. 2019. *SCORE: Assessment of your work setting safety, communication, operational reliability and engagement*. Duke University.

Singer, S., Meterko, M., Baker, L., et al. 2007. Workforce perceptions of hospital safety culture: Development and validation of the patient safety climate in healthcare organizations survey. *Health Services Research*, 42, 1999–2021.

Sorra, J. & Nieva, V. 2004. *Hospital survey on patient safety culture*. AHRQ Publication No. 04-0041. Agency for Healthcare Research and Quality.

Spurgeon, P., Sujan, M., Cross, S., et al. 2019. *Building safer healthcare systems*. Springer International Publishing.

Stanton, N. A., Salmon, P. M., Walker, G. H., et al. 2019. Models and methods for collision analysis: A comparison study based on the Uber collision with a pedestrian. *Safety Science*, 120, 117–128.

Sujan, M., Spurgeon, P. & Cooke, M. 2015. The role of dynamic trade-offs in creating safety – A qualitative study of handover across care boundaries in emergency care. *Reliability Engineering & System Safety*, 141, 54–62.

Vosper, H., Bowie, P. & Hignett, S. 2018. The NHS health check for developing HFE competencies. In: Charles, R. & Wilkinson, J. (eds.), *Contemporary ergonomics and human factors*. Chartered Institute of Ergonomics and Human Factors.

Waterson, P. 2014. *Patient safety culture: Theory, methods and applicaton*. CRC Press.

Westrum, R. 1993. Cultures with requisite imagination. In: Wise, J. A., Hopkin, V. D. & Stager, P. (eds.), *Verification and validation of complex systems: Human factors issues*. Springer Berlin Heidelberg.

Wiig, S., Aase, K., Billett, S., et al. 2020. Defining the boundaries and operational concepts of resilience in the resilience in healthcare research program. *BMC Health Services Research*, 20, 330.

Woods, D. D. & Hollnagel, E. 2006. Prologue: Resilience engineering concepts. In: Hollnagel, E., Woods, D. D. & Leveson, N. (eds.), *Resilience engineering: Concepts and precepts*. Ashgate.

CHAPTER 3

Tasks

Chapter Objectives and Learning Outcomes

- To describe the human contribution to task performance.
- To analyse systematically the impact of human performance on key vulnerabilities in the task.
- To reflect critically on the impact of work system and environmental factors on human performance.
- To assess the relative strengths and weaknesses of interventions aimed at improving human performance.

Introduction: Designing Tasks for Human Performance

A good starting point for analysing work systems is to look at what people are supposed to do (work-as-imagined), as well as what they actually do in practice (work-as-done), that is, their tasks. A thorough understanding of the tasks can then inform us about other elements of the work system, such as other tasks that have to be carried out, other people who are involved, the tools and the equipment that are going to be used, the physical spaces where the tasks are carried out, and the procedures, protocols and organisational structures that are in place. For now, we will consider these other elements of the work system in the form of generic factors that affect task performance, so-called performance-influencing factors (PIFs). Other chapters will then look at each of these elements in greater detail and provide guidance on how to improve the design and interaction of these work system elements.

This chapter describes a systematic approach for analysing people's tasks, and for identifying key vulnerabilities in these tasks in order to improve outcomes and everyone's well-being. The approach might help you, for example, with (see also Box 3.1):

- Addressing vulnerabilities identified in local incident investigations
- Implementing interventions suggested at national level to address known issues
- Investigating concerns raised by staff about vulnerabilities in their tasks
- Contributing to organisational development, quality improvement (QI) and process restructure projects.

BOX 3.1 Example – improving medicines reconciliation

> Reviews of patient safety incidents reported in a hospital identified a significant number of incidents relating to medications. The medicines reconciliation task is crucial to set the foundation for safe and effective care. If medicines reconciliation is not undertaken accurately or not undertaken at all, then this might result in potentially serious patient harm. A multi-professional team was set up to identify recommendations for improving the reliability and accuracy of this task in the hospital. The team analysed the task and identified several key vulnerabilities, such as failure to do medication reconciliation on admission, incorrect or incomplete transcription of medication onto the medication chart and providing an incomplete discharge letter. The team suggested improvements to address each of the identified vulnerabilities in the existing task set-up, but the main recommendation led to a task redesign including the introduction of an electronic medicines reconciliation system, which provided an improvement across several of the identified vulnerabilities in the task.

The overall approach is shown in Figure 3.1. In this chapter we will walk you through the steps of the approach, with a particular emphasis on two families of HF/E methods: 'task analysis' and 'human reliability analysis'. We describe a specific technique for each of these methods in greater detail.

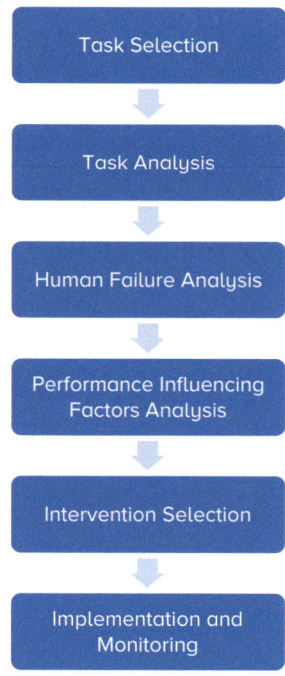

FIGURE 3.1 Systematic approach for analysing and improving human contribution to task performance.

Task Types

A task refers to goal-directed human activity, that is, something people do in order to achieve a goal. In everyday life this can be something mundane, such as making a coffee, or in health and social care settings this might be, for example, to arrange a GP appointment, to assess a patient, to request an x-ray or to undertake a home visit. A task typically has a clearly defined goal, as well as a start and end point. The notion of task is an analytical concept, and hence what we regard as the task for analysis depends on the scope of the analysis. For example, making a coffee might be the appropriate level of analysis, but, equally, to prepare dinner might be regarded as a suitable task and, therefore, level of analysis, if the analysis is concerned with an entire meal. In this instance, making a coffee would be a sub-task, maybe following the main meal. At times, you might start with a high-level task and realise that this is not the right level of analysis. In this case, you might wish to consider a lower-level task. For example, to manage patient flow in a hospital might be broken down into sub-tasks, and you could select a specific sub-task as the object of the task analysis, such as to prepare the discharge documentation for a patient. It depends on the focus of your analysis.

Tasks can be classified into different types. Some tasks have a predominantly physical aspect and are, accordingly, referred to as physical tasks. These are tasks where we can observe what is being done, for example the administration of drugs during the daily drug rounds. Other tasks, however, have a predominantly cognitive aspect, and we cannot easily observe what is going on. In these instances, we need to rely on people telling us what they are thinking in order to understand what they are doing. An example might be the interpretation of radiological images. These tasks are referred to as cognitive tasks. Lastly, there are tasks where teamwork and collaboration are important characteristics of the task. These are referred to as team (or collaborative) tasks. Emergency care provided to a trauma patient could be considered an example of a task where effective communication and collaboration between different members of the team are critical. Depending on the task type, different task analysis approaches might be more suitable than others.

Task Selection

The approach described in this chapter can be applied to analyse and improve a broad range of work situations. In practice, there are many tasks that could potentially be analysed, and some form of initial prioritisation needs to be carried out. It might be that a specific task has already been identified in a local incident investigation as requiring further analysis, or a national body might have suggested improvement interventions that require implementation at the local level. Having such an initial 'hook' can be helpful for ensuring buy-in and adequate organisational support. However, it is equally possible to use the approach for analysing tasks where there might have been concerns in the absence of adverse events or where there is a perceived need for greater clarity about how a task should be structured and carried out.

In order to focus the analysis, it is often useful to focus on tasks where the human contribution is particularly important or safety critical. For example, the vignette in Box 3.1 illustrates how a hospital team used incident investigations relating to medications to identify a broad area for improvement, and then selected medicines reconciliation as a particularly critical task, which they wanted to analyse further.

Studying Clinical Work Using Task Analysis

Task Analysis

If you want to improve clinical work and help people achieve their aims, it is important that you understand what people's aims are, how they go about achieving these aims and how the characteristics of their work might influence this. From a systems perspective, the aims are not the personal motivations of the individual, but represent the operational goals, such as transferring a patient from an ambulance to the emergency department, prescribing and administering medications, or requesting (and providing) an investigation. Task analysis (TA) is an HF/E framework or process that allows you to understand and represent what people do (or are supposed to do) in order to achieve the overall goals of the task, with a view to identifying problems and proposing potential improvements.

TA has been a cornerstone of HF/E for decades and is used in many different work contexts, including designing computer interfaces for air traffic controllers, ensuring safe staffing levels in control rooms in the nuclear and petrochemical industries, improving ambulance dispatch, reducing errors in maintenance tasks and many more. It is estimated that there over 100 different TA methods (Stanton et al., 2013). This large number of methods is due to several reasons. Each HF/E project might have a slightly different focus and aims, and hence methods were tailored to fit specific purposes. In addition, work and work systems have evolved considerably over the past 50 years, with the increasing introduction of automation, leading to greater emphasis on cognitive over manual work. This is reflected in a subcategory of TA methods with a specific focus on cognitive tasks, such as 'cognitive work analysis' (Vicente, 1999). However, at their core, all of the TA methods share a similar structure or process, which includes data collection of work tasks and their demands, representation in a format suitable for subsequent analysis, and then analysis of the tasks and the development of suggestions for improvement.

TA is frequently used in conjunction with other methods, which can either feed into the TA or which can use the TA as input for further analysis. Examples of the former include data collection methods, such as process walk-throughs or process maps; an example of the latter is the systematic identification and analysis of vulnerabilities, which we will describe in greater detail in this chapter.

Hierarchical Task Analysis

Hierarchical task analysis (HTA) is the most frequently used TA method, largely due to its universal applicability. HTA was developed in the late 1960s and early 1970s as a method to represent the broad range of human work activities, including some cognitive aspects, such as monitoring, anticipating and decision making (Stanton, 2006). HTA represents work based on a theory of goal-directed behaviour – this means it starts with the assumption that there is an overarching system or process goal, and that what people do is aimed at achieving this goal. HTA then structures what people do using a hierarchy of goals and sub-goals linked by plans, which describe how sub-goals combine to achieve the higher-level goal. Plans can be used to express any kind of algorithm, for example, simple sequential ordering (such as do step 1 to step 3 in order), free ordering (do steps 1, 2, 3 in any order), as well as more complex loops (such as do step 1 and step 2 in order until signal A is active, then do step 3). This representation creates a tree-like structure, where the leaves represent task steps that are considered elementary (for example, basic manual operations) or where further decomposition is not considered necessary.

Consider two examples to illustrate the workings of HTA. The first example is an everyday activity, in this case making a cup of tea (Figure 3.2). If we regard this as our goal, then we could say the essential sub-goals to achieve this might be (1) prepare materials, (2) brew tea, and (3) tailor to taste. Intuitively we know how to order these steps, but the plan can make this explicit: first prepare the materials, then brew the tea for one minute (say), and then tailor to your specific taste (for instance, by adding milk or sugar). It is also clear that we could further break down each of these goals in order to gain greater clarity about what is done. For example, preparation of materials could consist of fetching a cup, fetching a tea bag and placing the tea bag into the mug. When doing the HTA, it is advisable to start every step with a verb (for example, prepare, brew, tailor) and to avoid combinations of steps in a single task step; for example, you should avoid representing a step as 'prepare materials *and* brew tea'.

As a second example, consider giving an intravenous infusion of insulin. This is a more complicated task, and we will use it throughout this chapter. Our purpose with this example is to illustrate how the analysis works and, therefore, that the specific clinical

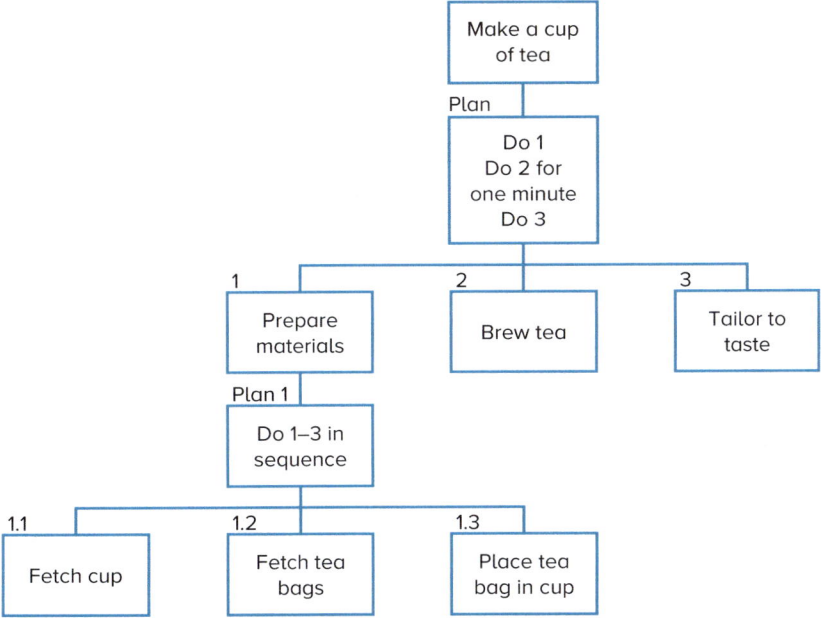

FIGURE 3.2 HTA representation for making a cup of tea.

details are not as important. The example is simplified, and we do not provide the full clinical context, so do not worry if there are clinical details that remain unclear. As a starting point, we could break down the overall goal into a number of sub-goals (Figure 3.3): check the prescription, prepare the syringe, prepare the infusion pump, do the cross checks, start the infusion, monitor the infusion, disconnect when the infusion is done and document the infusion. The plan indicates that steps 1–5 are to be carried out in order, and then step 6 (monitoring) will be undertaken until the infusion is complete. Only then, will steps 7 and 8 be carried out. Each of these steps could be broken down further.

To illustrate this iterative refinement, let us consider the preparation of the infusion pump (step 3) (Figure 3.4). This sub-goal involves several further activities: the

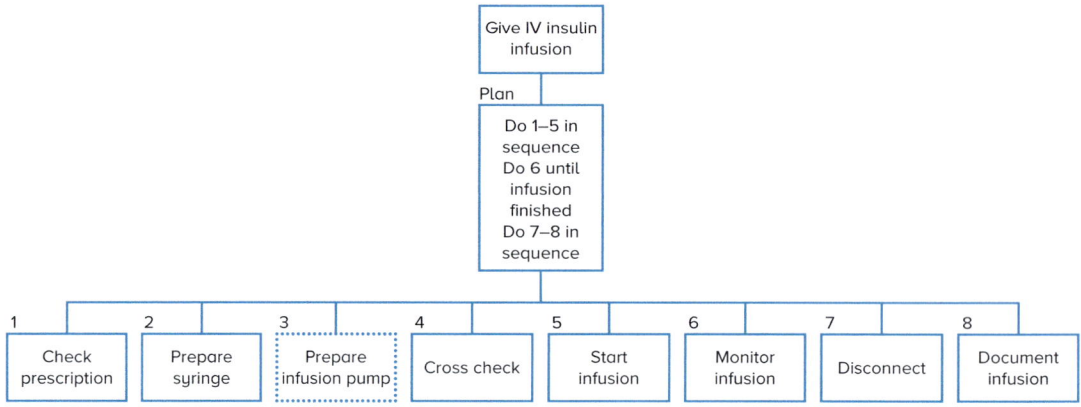

FIGURE 3.3 HTA for giving intravenous insulin infusion (high level).

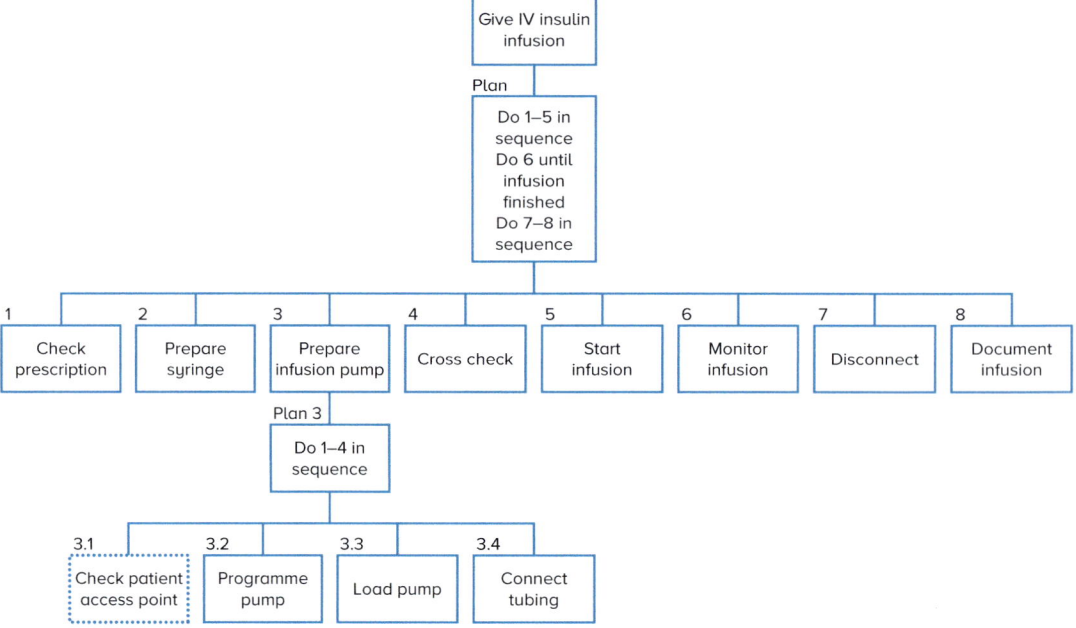

FIGURE 3.4 HTA for giving intravenous insulin infusion (first-level expansion).

nurse will check for a suitable patient access point (such as an existing line going into the patient to which the IV infusion can be connected), programme the pump, load the syringe into the pump and connect the tubing. These steps are done in sequence.

Again, we might wish to provide additional detail on these steps if there is value in analysing them further, for example, if it is known that certain steps are problematic or if there is a lack of clarity about how a step is carried out. In this case, we have analysed checking for an access point (step 3.1) further (Figure 3.5). The nurse needs to establish if there is a suitable access point in place and confirm that there are no signs of infection. In case there is no access point, or if an infection prevents its use, the nurse has to request a new IV access point. Once an access point is in place, the nurse checks that the IV device is patent and confirms that there are no contraindications for medications using the same access point.

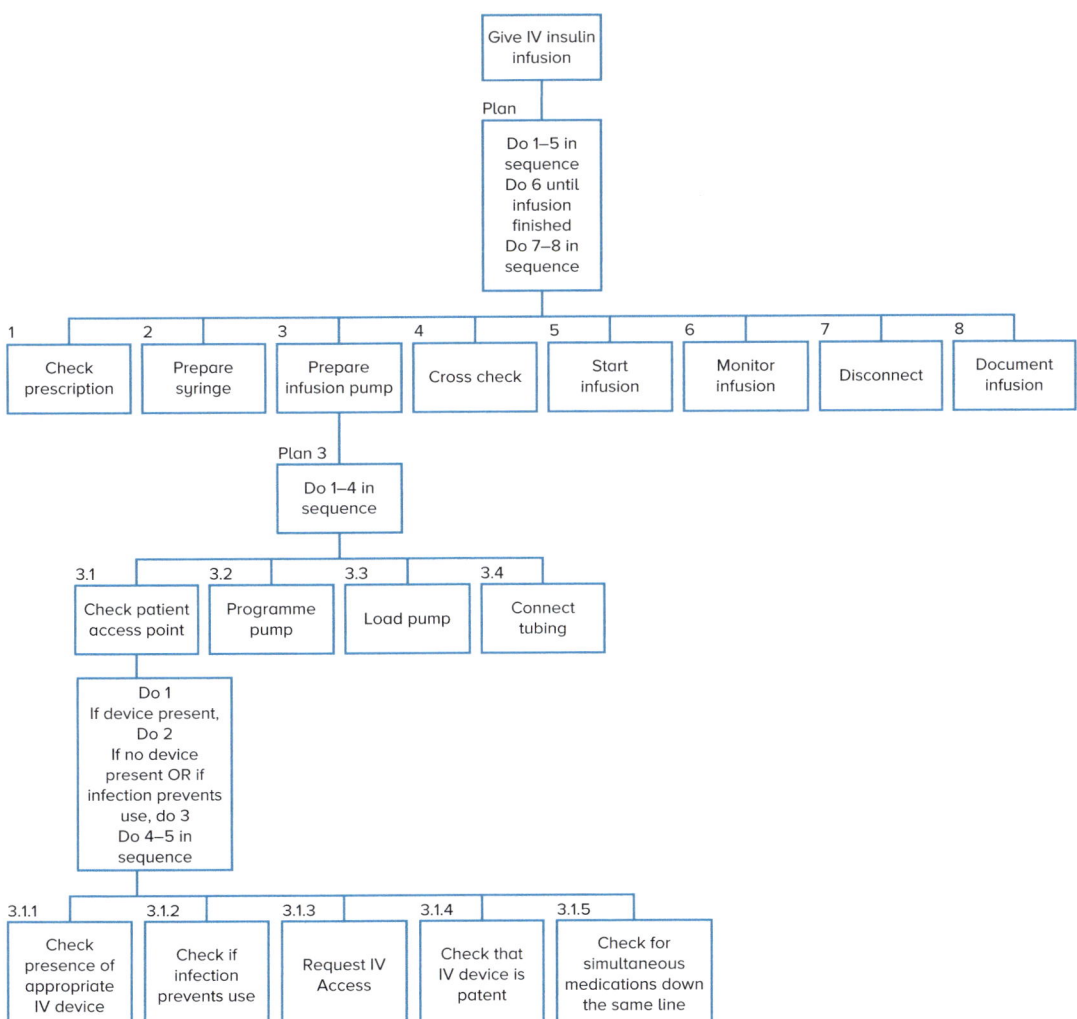

FIGURE 3.5 HTA for giving intravenous insulin infusion (second-level expansion).

At this point, we might determine that there is not much gained by breaking down these task steps further and consider some of the other higher-level steps in greater depth. There is no hard and firm stopping rule, and this decision is usually based on a number of criteria, such as purpose of the analysis, task complexity and availability of resources for doing the analysis.

Practical Considerations for Undertaking Task Analysis

In order to make TA and, more specifically, HTA work in practice, it is important to consider a few practical issues. It is helpful to have clarity about the purpose of the analysis. The examples demonstrate the very wide applicability of HTA, and there are many published examples available, including examples from healthcare (Chana et al., 2017; Lane et al., 2006; Parand et al., 2017). The main strengths of HTA are the flexible hierarchical decomposition, which allows activities to be broken down to the level that is considered adequate for the purpose of the analysis, and the explicit representation of algorithmic plans.

As mentioned above, a number of data collection approaches can feed into the TA or HTA. It is often useful to undertake some form of familiarisation with the task, for instance by doing process walks, observations and informal interviews. It is also advisable to identify and consider existing documentation, such as work procedures relevant to the task. It is not uncommon that the task itself is not documented in a single work procedure, but different steps might be covered by a broader range of procedures, guidelines or regulations. It is the job of the analyst to make sense of these and bring clarity to the task. HTA is well suited to support clinical teams in defining and understanding clinical processes, which hitherto had not been formally designed or documented.

The analyst can develop a preliminary TA based on this initial understanding of the task. The preliminary HTA (or other TA representation) is usually developed further and refined in focus groups with a small number of representative participants. If the task is fairly small and has a limited number of stakeholders (for example, just nurses), then one or two sessions with a few participants might be all that is required. On the other hand, if the task is larger and involves stakeholders from different departments or even different organisations (such as transfer of a patient from the ambulance service to the emergency department), then several sessions might be required. It is important that all relevant roles are involved, and that the focus groups allow for meaningful discussion.

The detail to which tasks are broken down depends on the purpose of the analysis, the complexity of the task and the importance of specific steps to successful task performance. It requires some experience with the method to get the level of breakdown right, because there is no exact stopping rule. If tasks are broken down into too much detail, then this requires a lot of effort, which could have been used more productively on other activities, such as analysing the critical steps using additional approaches.

The use of HTA can also provide team members from different backgrounds with the opportunity to build important relationships with each other, which in normal clinical practice they would not have. Creating opportunities to strengthen the social infrastructure of safety and enhancing staff engagement should be a key patient safety improvement strategy (Sujan, 2015).

Identifying Vulnerabilities in Clinical Tasks Using Structured Human Failure Analysis

Human Reliability Analysis

While the TA by itself is very useful for analysing and understanding clinical tasks, it can be helpful to apply additional, structured methods for systematically identifying vulnerabilities in the task. Such methods are known by different names, such as hazard analysis or risk analysis. In the HF/E literature, they are commonly referred to under the umbrella term 'human reliability analysis' (HRA).

HRA approaches were developed starting from the late 1960s and gained popularity during the 1980s in particular. The traditional aim of HRA techniques is to determine the impact of human error on a system. In a more modern interpretation, HRA techniques are used to reason systematically about human performance, the contextual conditions that impact human performance, and the improvements that can be put in place to improve overall system performance. The contextual conditions affecting human performance are the configurations of the work system and the interactions with other elements of the work system. For the purpose of the HRA they are typically referred to as 'performance-shaping factors' (PSF) or 'performance-influencing factors' (PIF).

There are over 75 documented HRA approaches. As with TA, this large number of different approaches is due to the fact that each might serve a slightly different purpose or focuses on a specific aspect. As many HRA approaches can also be used to provide quantitative estimates of human error probabilities, approaches vary in the underlying assumptions and methods for quantification, but we will consider only the qualitative use of HRA. This is because in practice the quantification of failures and their consequences can be extremely time consuming with a lot of uncertainty about the exact figures due to lack of relevant data. In most situations, a good qualitative understanding of potential failures is a sound basis for safety and quality improvement efforts, and this is the approach we recommend in this chapter.

In healthcare a variant of the prospective hazard analysis technique, 'failure modes and effects analysis' (FMEA), is a fairly well-known and well-established approach that can be used to identify and to analyse human errors (DeRosier et al., 2002). Increasingly, however, there are published examples of the use of traditional HRA approaches (that is, those developed in other industries) in healthcare (Sujan et al., 2020), such as SHERPA (see below), HEART, SPAR-H and CREAM (Chadwick and Fallon, 2012; Deeter and Rantanen, 2012; Phipps et al., 2008; Sands et al., 2015).

The Systematic Human Error Reduction and Prediction Approach

A technique for HRA that is generally regarded as reasonably easy to apply, while providing good reliability and validity, is the Systematic Human Error Reduction and Prediction Approach (SHERPA). SHERPA was originally developed to analyse and reduce errors in the nuclear and process industries, but has been used since in many other contexts (Embrey, 1986). It is similar in structure to FMEA, but it is based on a simple taxonomy of human errors, which can function as a guide for the identification of failure modes. SHERPA uses the HTA representation, and systematically analyses the basic task steps, that is, the bottom leaves in the HTA tree diagram. The analyst classifies each basic task step according to the behaviour type, and then applies the corresponding human error modes. The suggested behaviour types are action, checking, information retrieval, communication and selection. Basic human error modes for each of these behaviour types are shown in Table 3.1.

TABLE 3.1 SHERPA human error taxonomy

Behaviour type	Code	Error mode
Action	A01	Action too long/too short
	A02	Action mistimed
	A03	Action in wrong direction
	A04	Action too little/too much
	A05	Action too fast/too slow
	A06	Misalign
	A07	Right action on wrong object
	A08	Wrong action on right object
	A09	Action omitted
Checking	C01	Check omitted
	C02	Check incomplete
	C03	Right check on wrong object
	C04	Wrong check on right object
	C05	Check too early/too late
Information retrieval	R01	Information not obtained
	R02	Wrong information obtained
	R03	Information retrieval incomplete
	R04	Information incorrectly interpreted
Communication	I01	Information not communicated
	I02	Wrong information communicated
	I03	Information communication incomplete
	I04	Information communication unclear
Selection	S01	Selection omitted
	S02	Wrong selection

Chapter 3 Tasks

Once a credible human error mode has been applied, the analyst determines the potential consequences of this particular failure. Determining the potential consequences can be difficult, and it is often useful to think about both immediate consequences and more distal consequences. The next step is to consider whether there are any existing safeguards in place to prevent this failure from happening or to recover from it. If these are deemed insufficient, then the analyst can consider potential improvements.

Table 3.2 demonstrates the analysis for a part of the insulin infusion example. The analysis considers only the checking of the patient access point (step 3.1), which contains five sub-task (steps 3.1.1–3.1.5) and a corresponding plan, which describes the order in which the sub-tasks are to be carried out. Important steps are, for example, checking whether there are signs of access-site infection present, and checking for compatibility with other medications being giving via the same access point.

A credible error mode for checking for site infections is that this check is not carried out (Code C01 – Check omitted). If there is an infection, then this can become significantly worse from continued and additional use. The current risk controls rely on governance, training and staff competence. Performance-influencing factors include nurses undertaking concurrent activities and having high levels of workload. This can increase the likelihood that this check is forgotten. A potential intervention might be a reminder (or a compulsory check) via an electronic prescription and administration system.

Checking for compatibility with other medications is very important and safety critical. Potential error modes include not doing this check (Code C01 – Check omitted) or looking up the wrong medication from the different medications that the patient is on (Code C03 – Right check on wrong object). This can result in loss of potency of the drugs, potential toxicity, as well as several other serious adverse effects. The current risk control is the medication review at shift handover, where the medications the patient is on and the different access points are reviewed. Performance-influencing factors include concurrent activities, high workload, as well as the design of the work environment and the equipment. The work environment and equipment design can lead to situations where there are many different lines tangled up, and it might be hard to see easily which infusion is going through the different access points. Potential interventions might include an automated electronic compatibility check, as well as redesign of the work environment and equipment to avoid tangled lines.

Performance-Influencing Factors

As part of the analysis, you need to assess whether and how characteristics of the elements of the work system impact on the potential errors. HRA techniques typically include lists of performance-influencing factors (or performance-shaping factors) that you can use as prompts for an initial, quick assessment (Table 3.3). For example, if the task step involves using a piece of equipment, you might ask whether the usability (or lack of usability) affects task performance; you could check if work procedures are available, up to date and usable; and you could determine whether the physical environment has any impact on the task, for example noise and lighting. The lists

TABLE 3.2 Human failure and performance-influencing factors analysis example

Ref	Task type	Error type	Description	Consequence	Existing controls/ recovery	Performance-influencing factors	Recommended risk reduction
3.1 Check patient access point Plan 3.1 Do 1 If device present, do 2 If no device present OR if infections prevent use, do 3 Do 4–5 in sequence							
3.1.1 Check presence of appropriate IV device	Checking	C01 Check omitted	The nurse does not check that an IV device is present.	Delays are possible if there is no IV access, and the nurse will need to request one later.		Concurrent activities Workload	
3.1.2 Check if infection prevents use	Checking	C01 Check omitted	The nurse does not check for signs of site infection.	An existing site infection can become worse.	Relies on governance and training/ competence.	See 3.1.1	Include as required step in electronic prescription and administration system.

3.1.3 Request IV access	Communication	I01 Information not communicated	The nurse does not request a new IV access due to lack of suitably qualified colleagues available.	Delays in starting the infusion.		Staffing levels Workload	Provide training to ensure sufficient numbers of suitably qualified staff who can insert access points.
3.1.4 Check that IV device is patent	Checking	C01 Check omitted	The nurse does not check device patency.	Delays in giving the infusion.	The infusion pump will generate an alert based on detection of increased pressure.	Concurrent activities Workload	
3.1.5 Check for simultaneous medications down the same line	Checking	C01 Check omitted	The nurse does not check for other medications going down the same line.	Potential incompatibility of medications.	Review at shift change.	Concurrent activities Workload	Consider potential for automated checks.
		C03 Right check on wrong object	The nurse looks up the wrong medication.	See above.	See above.	Work environment (there can be many different and tangled lines with different access points) Equipment design Concurrent activities Workload	Consider potential for automated checks. Redesign of equipment and work environment.

TABLE 3.3 Examples of performance-influencing factors

Work system element	Example performance-influencing factors
Person	Physical capability and condition Fatigue Stress Workload Competence Quality of training Motivation Communication
Tasks	Complexity Unusual task Multi-tasking Distractions Time available Availability and quality of procedures
Tools and equipment	Usability Suitability Quality of interfaces Design Availability Maintenance
Physical spaces	Noise Heat Adequate space Lighting Ventilation Accessibility Clutter
Organisation	Work pressures Supervision Staffing levels Clarity of roles and responsibilities Safety culture Change management

serve as prompts, but it is advisable to assess performance-influencing factors via data collection techniques, such as observations and interviews.

Practical Considerations for Undertaking Human Reliability Analysis

The principles behind a SHERPA analysis are reasonably easy to understand, but doing a good human failure analysis can be challenging. The defining feature of failure analysis approaches is that they are systematic – they intend to provide us with a degree of confidence that we have looked at an issue in depth. Therefore,

Chapter 3 Tasks

lists of potential failure – or error – modes, such as the one provided in Table 3.1, are helpful. You should try and make use of these, and guard against jumping straight into what might look like the most important failures based on people's experience. Using the experience of people is clearly fundamental, but it needs to be carried out in a structured and systematic fashion, by going through each task step in turn, and thinking about potential failure modes. In this way, a broader range of situations and failures can be considered. This requires some discipline, and it is often helpful to have an experienced facilitator to keep the group on track.

Arguably, the biggest challenge in running human reliability assessments is the assessment of the consequences, especially when the method is used to create a quantitative output. In practice, we often find that the severity of the consequences is very much dependent on other factors, such as the patient's condition. If the patient is in a critical condition, then minor delays or deviations might result in death, whereas in a stable patient the severity of the consequences of the same failure might be negligible. It can be helpful to distinguish between immediate and more distal consequences, and to describe these qualitatively. For example, the immediate credible worst-case consequence of the failure to check if an infection prevents the use of an IV device (task step 3.1.2 in the example) might be that the IV device in an infected site continues to be used. The more distal consequence could be that the infection gets worse, which puts additional strain on the patient and could cause further complications, which require more explicit consideration from a clinician, thereby also increasing workload.

Intervention Selection

The TA and the human failure analysis provide a detailed understanding of the task and the current vulnerabilities. This can form the basis for designing and implementing appropriate interventions to reduce the vulnerabilities. The information provided by these approaches will not be the only consideration, but it can be a helpful starting point for creating a list of potential candidate interventions, which have transparent links to identified risks, and which can be appraised according to a range of criteria (for example, feasibility, affordability, level of risk reduction, ability to address multiple vulnerabilities with fewer interventions etc.).

When thinking about candidates for interventions, it is again a useful approach to do this systematically, rather than jumping straight to any specific intervention. For example, when double checks during medication administration are not carried out, it might be tempting to consider training and procedures as potential interventions. However, there might be other options. For example, it might be possible to include technology, such as barcodes, to reduce the risk of wrong medication administration. Of course, these can, in turn, introduce new vulnerabilities, which must be analysed and assessed.

In safety-critical industries a simple heuristic is commonly used to help people think about different types of candidate interventions in a systematic way. This so-called hierarchy of risk controls assumes that certain interventions are more effective at reducing risk than others. Accordingly, you should consider whether stronger risk controls are feasible before implementing weaker ones. Generally, the assumption is that it is better to eliminate risks where possible or to engineer safeguards that do not rely on people, before considering interventions that rely on people changing their behaviour or being more careful. So, for each identified risk, ask yourself:

- Can the risk or the source of the risk (the hazard) be eliminated?
- Can the reliance on people be reduced, for example, through automation?
- Can the performance-influencing factors be improved?

Only if the source of the risk cannot be eliminated, reliance on people cannot be reduced and the conditions within which people work have been optimised, then further behavioural risk controls could be considered, such as additional procedures, training, and reinforcement of messages around desirable behaviours (e.g., hand hygiene campaigns).

In practice, it is advisable to regard the hierarchy of risk controls as a helpful heuristic, but not as a static decision tool. The intention is to help the analyst to consider a range of options before selecting any specific intervention. In healthcare, the most frequently selected interventions tend to be at the bottom of the hierarchy of control, such as training, standardisation and formalisation of roles and responsibilities. However, this does not necessarily mean that these have to be ineffective, especially when they are done well (Liberati et al., 2018).

Consider the cross check in the insulin infusion example (task step 4). This is a critical check just before starting the infusion and is intended to be carried out by two nurses. However, potential failure modes are that either the check does not take place at all (Code C01 – Check omitted) or that only certain items are checked (Code C02 – Check incomplete). A potential engineering intervention could be the introduction of automated checks, which is something that is already included in many modern systems. Smart infusion pumps can check the drugs and the patient ID using barcode scanning, and the infusion activity can be mapped to the electronic prescribing system and compared against the prescription for any discrepancies. Potential interventions lower down the hierarchy of risk controls could include the introduction of a different type of pro forma, where nurses can tick off the different types of checks that have been done (thereby also serving as a memory aid and an audit tool). However, for both types of interventions it is important that (a) relevant stakeholders are involved in the design of the intervention, and (b) you consider potential new vulnerabilities that might be introduced with the intervention.

In addition, you can think about how to improve the performance-influencing factors. Excessive workload could be one reason why cross checks are not carried out, and this could be addressed through changes to staffing levels (which often is very difficult). The existing procedure might not reflect actual practice, and this could be updated and optimised, so that it provides greater flexibility and requires the most rigorous checks only for certain types of drugs.

Implementation and Monitoring

The outputs of the preceding steps are (a) a thorough understanding of the task and the main vulnerabilities, and (b) a set of candidate interventions that have clear links back to those vulnerabilities. This is very useful in order to enhance transparency of the overall process.

The next step is to implement the selected interventions. The detail of implementation is beyond the scope of this chapter, but it is helpful to bear in mind that interventions need to be monitored and their effectiveness reviewed. One way of doing this is to develop indicators for each intervention, which can be monitored over time. Lagging indicators are indicators that measure failures of risk control systems or interventions, which contributed to incidents and adverse events (for example, when reviewing incidents), while leading indicators measure the effectiveness of risk control systems during inspections and audits.

For example, if you were to introduce automated checks, then a lagging indicator might be the number of wrong medication administration incidents. A leading indicator for the automated checks could be routine audits to determine (a) the availability of the automated checking system (for example, whether it is physically available and working) and (b) the accuracy of the automated checks.

Chapter Summary

In this chapter you learnt about how to describe and analyse the tasks, which people undertake within clinical work systems. You were then introduced to a technique that allows you to identify and describe the main vulnerabilities in the task. You were sensitised to the potential impact of the quality of work system elements on successful task performance. You were presented with examples of different types of interventions. The approaches described in this chapter will enable you to critically reflect on how work is carried out and to create a transparent link between vulnerabilities and potential improvements, which can then be monitored and assessed over time.

CIEHF HF/E Competencies

Use of a human-centred approach to the design and development of systems
- Demonstrates ability to enhance health, safety, comfort, quality of life, attitudes, motivation, usability, effectiveness and efficiency.
- Understands the theoretical and practice bases for HF/E relating to design and development of systems.

Focus on how other system components and performance-influencing factors affect people
- Understands the theoretical and practice bases for analysis of human interactions.
- Understands the theoretical and practice bases for redesign of human interfaces.

Human capabilities and limitations
- Understands the theoretical and practice bases for HF/E relating to psychological and social capabilities and limitations.

Application of relevant methods, tools and techniques
- Understands the theoretical and practice bases for data collection and analysis relating to HF/E.

Professional skills and behaviours
- Understands role of HF/E in change strategies.

References

Chadwick, L. & Fallon, E. F. 2012. Human reliability assessment of a critical nursing task in a radiotherapy treatment process. *Applied Ergonomics*, 43, 89–97.

Chana, N., Porat, T., Whittlesea, C., et al. 2017. Improving specialist drug prescribing in primary care using task and error analysis: An observational study. *British Journal of General Practice*, 67, e157–e167.

Deeter, J. & Rantanen, E. 2012. Human reliability analysis in healthcare. *Proceedings of Symposium on Human Factors and Ergonomics in Health Care*. Human Factors and Ergonomics Society.

Derosier, J., Stalhandske, E., Bagian, J. P., et al. 2002. Using health care failure mode and effect analysis: The VA National Center for Patient Safety's prospective risk analysis system. *Joint Commission Journal on Quality Improvement*, 28, 248–267, 209.

Embrey, D. 1986. SHERPA: A systematic human error reduction and prediction approach. *Proceedings of the International Topical Meeting on Advances in Human Factors in Nuclear Power Systems.* American Nuclear Society.

Lane, R., Stanton, N. A. & Harrison, D., 2006. Applying hierarchical task analysis to medication administration errors. *Applied Ergonomics*, 37, 669–679.

Liberati, E. G., Peerally, M. F. & Dixon-Woods, M. 2018. Learning from high risk industries may not be straightforward: A qualitative study of the hierarchy of risk controls approach in healthcare. *International Journal for Quality in Health Care*, 30, 39–43.

Parand, A., Faiella, G., Franklin, B. D., et al. 2017. A prospective risk assessment of informal carers' medication administration errors within the domiciliary setting. *Ergonomics*, 61, 104–121.

Phipps, D., Meakin, G. H., Beatty, P. C., et al. 2008. Human factors in anaesthetic practice: Insights from a task analysis. *British Journal of Anaesthesia*, 100, 333–343.

Sands, G., Fallon, E. F. & van der Putten, W. J. 2015. The utilisation of probabilistic risk assessment in radiation oncology. *Procedia Manufacturing*, 3, 250–257.

Stanton, N. 2006. Hierarchical task analysis: Developments, applications, and extensions. *Applied Ergonomics*, 37, 55–79.

Stanton, N., Salmon, P. M., Rafferty, L. A., et al. 2013. *Human factors methods: A practical guide for engineering and design*. Ashgate.

Sujan, M. 2015. An organisation without a memory: A qualitative study of hospital staff perceptions on reporting and organisational learning for patient safety. *Reliability Engineering & System Safety*, 144, 45–52.

Sujan, M. A., Embrey, D. & Huang, H. 2020. On the application of Human Reliability Analysis in healthcare: Opportunities and challenges. *Reliability Engineering & System Safety*, 194, 106189.

Vicente, K. J. 1999. *Cognitive work analysis: Toward safe, productive, and healthy computer-based work*. CRC Press.

CHAPTER 4

The People

Chapter Objectives and Learning Outcomes

- To describe human capability and its relationship with tasks, tools and the environment.
- To understand the importance of designing tasks and work environments in a way that takes into account the full range of capabilities and human performance.
- To explore ways in which you might better understand workforce and patient or service-user capabilities.

Introduction: Understanding the Capabilities of the People Working Within Your System

We have already considered the importance of task design in supporting human performance and looked at some of the factors that may shape or influence this performance. It is now time to look at this in a little more detail. When we take an HF/E approach to understanding work tasks, we are really asking the following:

- Can *this* person (worker, team, patient, etc.) ...
- With *this* training (or information) ...
- Do *this* task ...
- With *this* equipment (or service) ...
- To *these* standards (performance) ...
- Under *these* conditions?

We also want to know whether they can achieve this level of performance repeatedly, as these tasks are likely to be done many times over. Task performance depends on the interaction between the person, the task and any tools and technologies they may use, and cannot be separated from the context in which this happens. A particularly important relationship is that between the demands exerted by the task and the capabilities of the person.

This chapter might be of particular use for:

- Proactive evaluation of tasks, hazards and the potential for failure
- Incident investigation

Human Factors and Ergonomics in Health and Social Care

- Designing new procedures, processes and tools
- Procurement.

Match of Human Capabilities to Tasks

Throughout this book, we talk about the centrality of design to HF/E. According to Pheasant and Haslegrave (2006, p. 5):

> [If intended for human use,] design should be based on the physical and mental characteristics of its human users (insomuch as these may be determined by the investigative methods of the empirical sciences).

The aim is to fit the equipment (or task) to the user, not the user to the equipment or task. Any equipment or task should be designed to allow the user to be productive, but they should also be able to use the equipment (or complete the task) easily, comfortably and safely. We have mentioned that when a person interacts with tasks and equipment, they do so in a specific context, and this has to be considered. If we take the example of taking blood pressure manually (Box 4.1), we need to consider

BOX 4.1 The demands of a specific task – manual blood pressure management

The demands of a task can change depending on the interactions of the elements of a work system, e.g., when different tools are used, or the task is carried out in different physical spaces. Task demands need to match human capabilities and characteristics.

Consider the task of manual measurement of blood pressure. It is worth considering that manual measurement is still the 'gold standard', despite an increasing shift towards using electronic devices. Manual measurement (especially using the old mercury sphygmomanometer) reflects pressure changes in the cuff directly driven by the presence or absence of blood flow through the artery. Electronic devices instead measure volume changes in the cuff, which are interpreted via an algorithm built into the software.

So what is behind the move to electronic blood pressure measurement? Manual blood pressure measurement is quite a difficult task to learn and to get right all the time. This is partly because of the design of the equipment – a lack of standardisation of the equipment (particularly the cuff) can make it hard to set the task up correctly, and quite a high degree of dexterity and co-ordination is required to handle the equipment, exerting significant motor demands on the user. It also exerts significant visual demands (the user needs to be able to read the measurement) and aural demands. These latter demands can be particularly influenced by the environment. If the lighting is poor, or there is glare from a window, it may be hard to read the scale. Similarly, accurate measurement of the pressure requires the user to hear Korotkoff sounds – noisy environments make this challenging. Success, however, will not just depend on the equipment and environmental demands, but on the user's visual, aural, cognitive and motor capabilities, and whether these are adequate to meet the demands.

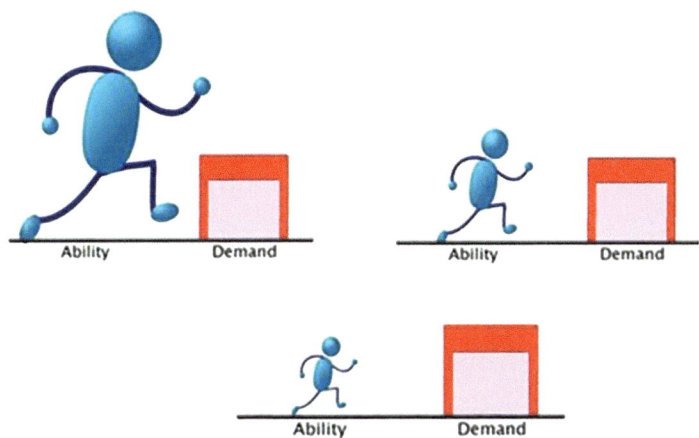

FIGURE 4.1 Success in a task requires that the user's capabilities can meet the demands exerted by the task.

things like the ambient noise and the availability (or not) of other pieces of equipment within the environment. We also have to consider the users and their capabilities.

If you consider Figure 4.1, you can perhaps appreciate that if the capabilities of the user far exceed the demands exerted by the task, then there will be no problem – the task can be completed easily. If the imbalance is the other way round, and the demands of the task far exceed the capabilities of the user, then it will be impossible to do the task. A third (and common) possibility is the situation where the user's capabilities just about meet the demands of the task. In this situation, it is possible that the task will be completed satisfactorily, but you can appreciate that under certain circumstances where either the demands of the task increase or the capabilities of the user are reduced, the quality of the task may reduce, or it may even become impossible.

Task demands may increase for many reasons. A common one is the fact that tasks tend to be designed as though they will be the only task carried out by the user. In reality, workers are likely to have to cope with multiple tasks at the same time. Unforeseen factors, such as the breakdown of equipment, or increased pressures from management or policies, may all increase demands. Individual capabilities vary on a daily basis – a worker may be nearing the end of a 12-hour shift and be fatigued or anxious to complete all the required tasks and provide a comprehensive handover. Perhaps their eyesight is not great; it is fine when they are completing the task in a brightly lit area, but as the light dims, they are unable to adapt. Intelligent task design minimises the task demands, accepts people may work when fatigued, stressed or compromised, and maximises user capability in all these scenarios. This should help you to see that HF/E requires not only an understanding of the whole system (and where this system fits into other systems), but also an understanding of the tasks within that system and their demands. You also need to know who your users (people using or experiencing the system) are, what is expected of them, the contexts they are required to work in, and their capabilities.

So, in short, capability–demand theory requires you to consider:

- Who your users are
- What tasks they are undertaking
- The tools at their disposal
- Their capabilities
- The context (environment) in which the tasks take place
- What demands the task and the tools make on the user
- How these may be influenced by environment
- Whether there is a mismatch between capability and demand.

Performance-Influencing Factors

Recognising human capabilities and optimising human performance is a key principle for human factors professionals. This requires an understanding of how the design of the system, tasks and organisational culture can create working conditions that enhance or challenge human physical or cognitive capabilities. In Chapter 3 we described the Systematic Human Error Reduction and Prediction Approach (SHERPA), which systematically considers the nature of tasks and the potential or reported failures, and identifies performance-influencing factors (PIFs) (that may have been identified as likely to have impacted the outcome. Typically, human factors practitioners will consider the scientific evidence to understand how the relevant PIF may influence human performance. Human factors practitioners often start by understanding what is required of the person to complete the task and how the task may be vulnerable to failure (Chartered Institute of Ergonomics and Human Factors, 2023). For example, tasks that require focus of attention to information to enable judgements and decisions to be made may be vulnerable to a person's level of fatigue, experience, the quality of the information presented and distractions or time available to them. Tasks that require communication may be vulnerable to noise in the environment or the need for face masks. These examples indicate how a full understanding of the nature of tasks, the environments in which they are completed and the equipment used can help to anticipate how people performing the tasks may be impacted. There are many potential lists of PIFs; the key is to ensure the stages of the tasks are linked to relevant PIFs. Some PIFs may be generic across all tasks, such as distractions or noise, and this could be stated in a summary of your analysis. We will consider three frequently reported PIFs below (Figure 4.2) to illustrate how and why these may be relevant to health and social care settings and to suggest how further evaluation could be achieved.

Workload

Workload is a concept much studied in the field of human factors, with little consensus on how best to measure its impact (Young et al., 2014). We can consider workload on a spectrum, ranging from high to low, with both ends of the spectrum relevant to understand the reliability and quality of work performance. Workload may refer to problems or questions raised around different levels of demand, associated with the number or complexity of tasks, how many staff are required to manage a

Chapter 4 The People

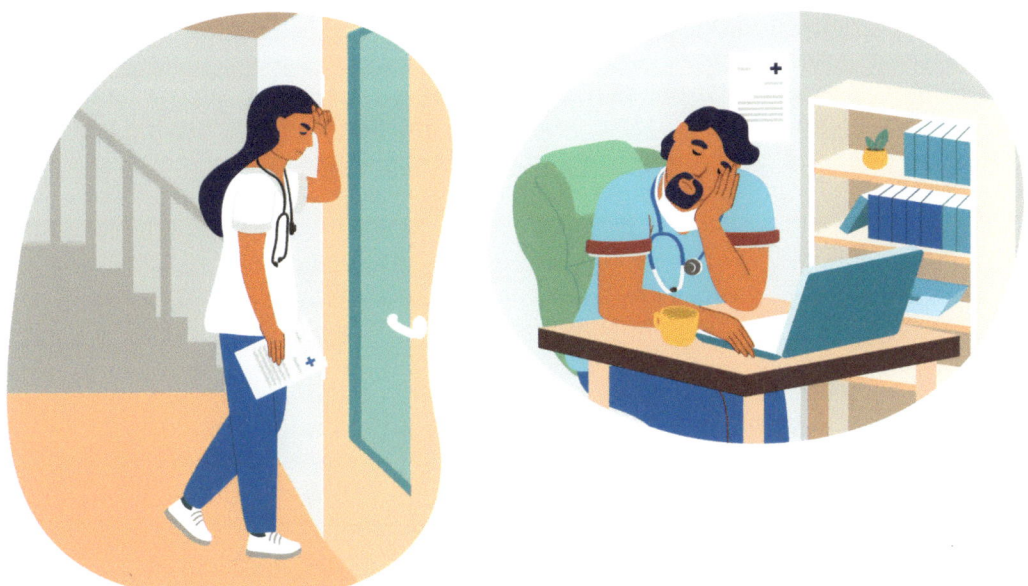

FIGURE 4.2 Performance-influencing factors, such as workload, fatigue and stress, impact on human performance.

Source: Shutterstock/Siberian Art.

specific number of patients or service users, or the skill mix required to ensure the workload across a team promotes a high level of quality in the care provided. The term workload should also consider the response to the demand associated with work; this refers to the effort perceived or associated by staff to accommodate the demand from the work required. The associated effort will be influenced by the level of demand but also an individual's experience, cognitive capabilities, expected level of performance, the time available to complete the work, and even the time of day.

The two examples described in Box 4.2 suggest that if we wish to measure workload and understand how high and low levels may influence performance and reliability in these workplaces, different approaches to workload assessment would be necessary. To consider the impact of workload first requires insight into the task and the context of the work completed by a particular staff group.

The organisational context can make even a simple task a workload challenge, as workload is not solely about human capabilities and the properties of a task, but also the individual's interaction with the environment and organisational pressures. The calculation of a medication dose could be simple arithmetic; writing or inputting this into a medical record can be a simple transcription task. In the context of a ward doctor or pharmacist completing this at the end of a 12-hour shift, on a ward with multiple interruptions and distractions, with the pressure to discharge patients quickly to ensure the flow of patients through the hospital, these interactions may create high levels of workload experienced by the individual. This may influence the time required to achieve all tasks, as other tasks may be shed to prioritise the task that the person is being chased to do. The context can increase the level of workload

BOX 4.2 Cognitive and physical workload examples

A radiologist's workload requires high levels of vigilance when undertaking thousands of scans to identify abnormalities. This task demands high levels of sustained attention to ensure high reliability. To the outside observer this may look like a task that could be categorised as having a low level of workload. However, there is a high level of mental workload required to sustain a high level of attention. It is well recognised there is a deterioration in sustained attention after 15–20 minutes. Task reliability becomes vulnerable, and strategies are required to refocus mental attentional resources.

How work is designed, moving between tasks with different mental demands, acknowledging limitations of human attention and designing technology to assist with tasks that we know humans may struggle to complete over long periods of time or repetitively, are all ways to manage this type of workload.

Considering the workload of a porter, it may be the physical demands that challenge human capabilities, and without effective management of workloads, high levels of work-related injuries may occur. Mitigating for awkward postures or repetitive high loading can be achieved through the use of assistive devices or by rotating between jobs with differing physical workloads.

experienced and influence how trade-offs or adjustments may affect practices and reduce the effectiveness of organisational policies and standards.

Job design, rotation of roles and designing workplaces and equipment to acknowledge the impact of the associated workload should be considered as part of a systems-based mindset for improving the quality and safety of care. To manage workload as a system risk requires an understanding of tasks, as described in Chapter 3, alongside processes for the evaluation of workload.

Methods to understand tasks are well established and transferable to health and social care (see Chapter 3). The evaluation of workload is less well established in health and social care compared to other industries; however, there are a few examples (Hoonakker et al., 2011; Tully et al., 2021). There are some general principles for the measurement of workload. These include the fact that workload is multi-dimensional and, therefore, requires a need for both subjective and objective measures. Subjective measures reflect staff perceptions of the associated effort and demand of a single task or set of tasks: for example, 'On a scale of one to ten, how much effort do you exert to complete this task?' Objective measurement refers to something that can be observed or recorded, and then considered to reflect demand on a person: for example, the duration, physical effort or cognitive demand of a task. Objective measures of workload are based on the assumption that the demand from work will create a physiological response to accommodate it. The type of response will be dependent upon the type of task but might include heart rate, pupil dilation and sweat responses (Charles and Nixon, 2019). Physiological measures can be valuable in combination with subjective perceptions; however, infection protection control restrictions, such as bare below the elbow, can limit healthcare staff wearing watches to collect physiological metrics. There are other measures that seek to capture characteristics of operational demand specific to a work setting. These may act as an indirect measure if they capture task demands recognised as being correlated to staff workload, for example, wait times, error rates and the ability to complete additional secondary or low priority tasks, and are triangulated with other workload measures.

Finally, there are differences in measures intended to reflect physical workload and cognitive workload. Although there are no ready-made tools for every type of job role in health and social care, Table 4.1 highlights a few subjective workload tools developed by other industries that could be tried or modified when looking to understand workload in health and social care settings. Box 4.3 illustrates examples of workload assessment in healthcare. However, these tools should be approached

TABLE 4.1 Common workload assessment methods

Workload measures	References	Description
NASA-TLX (Task Load Index)	Hart and Staveland (1988)	A multi-dimensional rating procedure to provide an overall score of workload. This scale has six subscales: mental demands, physical demands, temporal demands, own performance, effort and frustration. Each dimension is assigned a relative weight based on pair-wise comparison. Then a rating (0–100) is assigned to each dimension and combined with the previously assigned weight to calculate an overall score.
RawTLX	Hart (2006)	A modification of the original NASA-TLX. The scores from each dimension are added and averaged, rather than assigned individual weights (that is, their influence is assumed to be equal).
SWAT (Subjective Workload Assessment Technique)	Reid and Nygren (1988)	SWAT is based on three dimensions of workload: time load, mental effort load and psychological stress load. Each dimension is divided into three points (1–3) for scoring.
IWS (Integrated Workload Scale)	Pickup et al. (2005)	IWS is intended to support staff to estimate their perceived workload in real time. The person is prompted at regular intervals to give a rating on a scale and to reflect a snapshot of time relative to tasks or operational situation. A 9-point rating scale is used, ranging from 'not demanding' to 'too demanding'.

cautiously, as they are not without controversy. A cautionary note is therefore offered in selecting tools and certain considerations are needed: what is the aim of the evaluation; does the tool makes sense in the context and to those required to use it; and will any information gathered better inform you of the risk of either the physical or cognitive workload? A mix of objective and subjective measures is usually the preferred approach to developing a profile representing the workload of a predefined context or workplace.

Stress

Stress has been defined as 'the adverse reaction people have to excessive pressures or other types of demand placed on them' (Health and Safety Executive, n.d.). It is a

BOX 4.3 Examples of workload assessment in healthcare

RawTLX
Hoonakker et al. (2011) used NASA-TLX to evaluate workload as experienced by 757 intensive care nurses across 21 units. This study was intended to evaluate the validity of the tool, RawTLX, for assessing nursing staff workload. They collected ratings and compared these to a number of variables: nurses' age, showing little difference; duration of shift, indicating 12-hour shifts rated higher (that is, higher workload) than 8-hour shifts; and comparisons across eight hospital sites, highlighting that workload was rated higher in the larger sites. The authors compared the ratings to operational characteristics, such as nurse–patient ratio, which interestingly did not correlate with the workload rating scale. The study concludes that RawTLX has validity and reliability in this context and offers a possibility to understand subjective levels of workload in healthcare.

NASA-TLX and SWAT
NASA-TLX and SWAT are the most frequently used workload tools; Huggins and Claudio (2018) compared their use in the context of a cancer care clinic. They used both tools to evaluate the workload associated with preparing and delivering treatment, checking on patients and cleaning the clinical area, and administrative work with computers. This study suggested that the majority of the dimensions in the NASA-TLX correlated with those within SWAT, except for the dimensions of performance and frustration, which the NASA-TLX scale alone captured.

Integrated Workload Scale
Taking time to complete subjective scales with multiple dimensions is not always possible in the context of work environments. This has led to the development of tools that can be applied to gain instantaneous ratings. The IWS was used by Tully et al. (2021) to understand the optimal time to introduce a sign-out from a theatre session. The IWS was used to collect workload ratings of individual roles within a theatre team at different points. This illustrated high variability and unequal workloads across the team, and the use of direct observations and workload ratings supported the co-design and implementation of timing and roles most suited to leading the sign-out process.

concept that has consequences for how well a person may cope with their workload or work context, and ultimately it has huge implications for an organisation in terms of the sustainability of a sufficient and effective number of staff to deliver a service. This highlights the significance for an organisation to evaluate and understand the nature of workload and the consequence of stress in health and social care settings, as stress becomes one of the greatest costs to organisations due to staff absences or resignations and the consequent need to backfill staff. Stress is a consequence of the interaction of people with other elements of their work system in their environment. Although individual personality differences may influence how we personally manage stress, it is the control we have in any given context that will determine the individual experience. This is recognised as having implications for patient safety, the productivity of staff and the quality of their care for patients (Carayon et al., 2014). Engaging staff in a systems approach using the Systems Engineering Initiative for Patient Safety (SEIPS) to explore their perceptions of their workplace and workload can help understand key local stressors and support consideration of how to enable greater control in their management through co-design of action plans.

Health and social care in the UK face a well-documented challenge from the impact of stress on staff and the provision of a sufficient workforce to manage demand for services. A useful summary and practical tools to reflect the current situation is provided by West (2021), with a call for the need for compassion in the leadership of health and social care to manage the future challenges.

Fatigue

Fatigue is a consequence of a reduction in quality sleep, reduced number of hours slept or sleep deprivation from extended periods of wakefulness (Kayser et al., 2022). Fatigue is a physiological state created due to workload or working against circadian rhythms (the timing of an individual's biological clock within the brain), with recognised effects on both cognitive and physical performance of tasks (Gurubhagavatula et al., 2021). Degradation in cognitive performance includes slow response times, increased lapses in attention, reduced reliability in switching between tasks and reduced ability to reliably recall, manipulate and apply information to solve problems (Kayser et al., 2022).

The concept of staff fatigue is rarely managed as an organisational risk within health or social care, and it is a risk to patient or service-user safety. The duration of shifts, shift patterns and the opportunity or facilities to rest between and within shifts are all factors influential to cumulative staff fatigue. Fatigue is very much influenced by the organisation's view of their responsibility to consider fatigue as a risk to well-being and safety.

The impact of fatigue is well evidenced as being detrimental to fine motor control, working memory and decision making, increasing risk-taking behaviours and contributing to an incremental increase in errors noted beyond the duration of an eight-hour shift or a greater number of consecutive shifts (Folkard and Lombardi, 2004; Salminen, 2010). There is some evidence of direct links to staff or patient safety events (Gurubhagavatula et al., 2021; Kayser et al., 2022); however, as with all other industries, it is not always easy to clearly identify fatigue as the cause of an incident, although evidence can be collected to consider its likely contribution. A few factors to consider might be how much sleep has been obtained prior to a shift. The first night shift is recognised as a risk factor, as sleep prior to the shift can often be challenging. Prolonged wakefulness can create fatigue, with the evidence acknowledging that after 16–17 hours awake, staff will be working (or driving home) with reactions equivalent to those of a person at the legal drink–drive alcohol limit (Williamson and Feyer, 2000). As a rule of thumb, for every hour of sleep you will gain two hours of alertness at work (Dawson and McCulloch, 2005).

The duration and pattern in the rotation of shifts can highlight a greater risk for fatigue. Also important is the culture or local team climate that determines attitudes towards taking a break to enable rest, or time for and access to food and drink. The concept of fatigue management programmes (Box 4.4) is starting to be looked at in healthcare and is worth reading about to consider in the context of patient safety (Dawson and McCulloch, 2005; HSSIB, 2024). Even if an entire programme cannot immediately be embedded, a level of risk awareness can commence; patient safety leads can introduce the risks of fatigue to healthcare staff, and the organisation can enter fatigue onto their risk register to promote a need for actions to manage the associated risks (Association of Anaesthetists, 2023).

BOX 4.4   Examples of key approaches for fatigue risk management programmes

Fatigue risk management can be considered from three perspectives:

Predictively – to anticipate fatigue-inducing conditions for specific job roles and to understand the implications for fatigue when modifying work practices. An organisation can consider and act upon factors known to impact sleep and fatigue, such as working hours, the opportunity to rest, rostering and biomathematical modelling of shift patterns.

Proactively – to monitor, measure and manage fatigue levels as a consequence of current work design. This may require an organisational strategy and policy to outline where and how this should be achieved, roles to oversee the management of risks, education on fatigue and provision of the facilities to enable rest, as well as systematic collection and analysis of data to reflect work hours, shift patterns worked and data or enquiries to reflect performance and incidents rates that may indicate the impact of fatigue.

Reactively – to provide organisational learning to identify the need to respond to the impact of fatigue. Incident investigations that consider fatigue as a potential contributory factor and collate shifts and data to reflect workload and the opportunity to rest and recover. Audits and reviews of sickness, absence, staff retention and occupational health referrals that may indicate fatigue as a source of concern to individuals and organisational performance.

Designing to Meet Human Characteristics – Inclusive Design

Identifying Your Users

When we talk about 'users', we are not referring to a homogeneous group of people; if we consider a piece of equipment, we may initially only think about patients or service users and the frontline staff who have to use it as part of their job. However, others will have to procure it, maintain, repair, clean and store it, and still others will have to write standard operating procedures (SOPs) to support its use. The same goes for environments and tasks; we need to consider all the people who will be interacting with these elements of the work system. This rarely happens in practice, and most probably reflects an absence of systems thinking. While we have chosen SEIPS as our model for this book, sometimes a criticism levelled against it as a tool is that it doesn't necessarily encourage users to think outside the organisation (or even organisational unit) when looking for factors that influence performance. Although this is technically covered in SEIPS through the 'external environment' work element, without additional guidance it is perhaps difficult to apply in practice.

Defining User Capabilities

When a person uses a piece of equipment, it exerts demands on them. These demands may be physical, such as requiring strength or co-ordination. They might require the user to be able to see or hear information, and it will also exert cognitive demands, as the person will have to understand how to use it. The user meets these demands (or tries to) with their capabilities. Capabilities include:

- Visual (acuity, contrast sensitivity, field of view, stereopsis)
- Hearing (ability to detect pure tones, speech, location)
- Motor (reach, grip, linear and rotational strength, endurance, co-ordination, precision)
- Language
- 'Handedness'
- Neurodiversity
- Cognitive (information perception, alertness and attention, comparison with 'stored info' – mix of long-term and short-term memory necessary for 'prospective memory').

It is important to realise that capabilities (i) are highly variable within the population, (ii) almost invariably decline with age and (iii) can also be significantly impacted by ill health and factors influencing our physiology, such as nutrition, hydration, fatigue or stress. Remember that we do not only have an ageing patient population, but also an ageing workforce. It is also important to consider that the equipment is used in a specific context, which may change – our noisy environment is a good example. We might be able to use the manual sphygmomanometer successfully in a quiet environment, but if the noise level increases too much, we might not be able to hear well enough to use the instrument effectively. Similarly, standardisation of equipment is rare in healthcare, and equipment may change at short notice – an unfamiliar bit of kit would exert increased cognitive demands. Capability may change; perhaps you've left your glasses at home and now you can't read the information on the equipment, or perhaps you are feeling unwell and cognitive function is a bit below par. From a quality and safety perspective, we ideally want to make equipment selections that ensure demands are fewer than capabilities for all users (or at least most users), and recognise that users may not always be in tip top condition (for instance, they may be tired or hungry). This means we need to work with the users to understand their capabilities, and design equipment and tasks to acknowledge and accommodate these limitations.

Designing for Inclusion

Anthropometry is the measurement of the physical properties of the human body. It includes things such as stature (height), girth, shoulder breadth and reach range. It also includes grip strength and measurements of things such as visual acuity. It is clear that in many ways anthropometric measurements reflect physical aspects of capability. Chapter 6 (on Environment) provides examples of methods used to consider anthropometric dimensions and the potential for injury. Such measurements are usually normally distributed within the population, so can be represented by the bell-shaped curve shown in Figure 4.3. For such distributions, values falling within two standard deviations from the mean account for 97.7% of the total. This data is used in different ways in design. For inclusive designs, we want as many people as possible to be able to use our product. For example, if you think about a door, it has an important safety aspect to it – you need everyone to be able to get through it in an emergency. The important anthropometric measurements here would be stature and probably hip and shoulder width. You would consider the mean measurement and then probably adjust this to accommodate those on the 99.999th percentile. However, sometimes we want to design in the opposite direction; for example, we might want to prevent people from getting their head stuck in railings, so we might design to include only the 0.001th percentile, meaning that the vast majority of people would be unable to get their heads through the gaps in the railings.

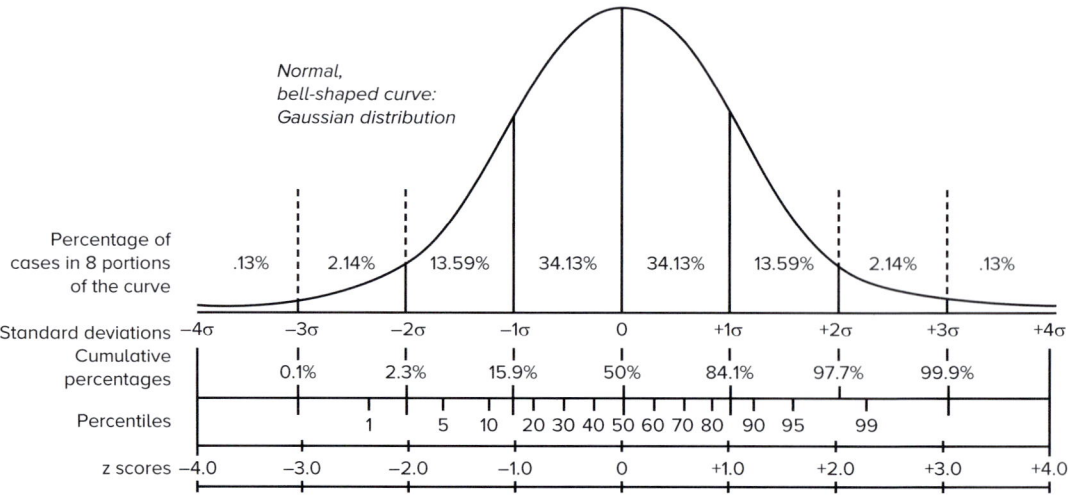

FIGURE 4.3 Most anthropometric measurements are normally distributed.

Inadvertent Exclusion

A study by Ward et al. (2010) took a systems approach to exploring methotrexate toxicity. Regular occurrences of inadvertent overdose led to a series of National Patient Safety Alerts. They used a safety analysis method called Hazard and Operability Studies (HAZOP) (Box 4.5) to identify the highest risk scenarios relating to methotrexate administration. Three of these involved packaging and labelling:

- At home: Confusing 2.5 mg and 10 mg tablets
- At home: Taking methotrexate instead of folic acid
- In the pharmacy: Picking error (10 mg instead of 2.5 mg).

To unpack this, researchers worked with patients and directly observed them taking medication at home. This revealed that designing for exclusion (in the form of childproof packaging) had the inadvertent effect of excluding arthritis patients from their medication. Elderly patients whose capabilities were further reduced by the nature of their condition struggled to remove their medication from a childproof bottle, so they worked round this by decanting tablets into other storage containers, which were not only no longer childproof, but also potentially impacted on drug stability, as the tablets were no longer in an airtight pack. Most importantly, because of the similarities in the appearance of methotrexate (to be taken once weekly) and folic acid (to be taken daily), it runs the risk of confusion and can result in methotrexate overdose.

A common form of exclusion is that of wheelchair users accessing buildings or toilets. This may be in the case of public buildings or healthcare settings. Doorways that are too narrow may not accommodate both the breadth of a wheelchair and the user's

BOX 4.5 Hazard and Operability Studies

HAZOP (Hazard and Operability Studies) is a systematic approach to identifying and describing risks in a process. It considers the process as it happens in a specific context by involving relevant workers. It has a long history in chemical industries, but also the energy sector and pharmaceutical manufacturing. It begins with a process map (which, in the case of these other sectors, is usually a map of the equipment involved, often referred to as 'piping and instrumentation diagrams'). These diagrams or process maps are built with input from those working across the system to ensure that they are accurate enough for the next stage, which is a form of risk analysis. Guide words are used to anticipate ways in which various functions might deviate from what is planned. For example, you could imagine that in piping diagrams, flow might be an issue. Guide words might therefore include 'no', 'reduced' or 'more' flow.

HAZOP is a qualitative approach, based on the assumption that failures are caused by deviation from an ideal designed process. It does not, by itself, produce quantitative estimates of risk, but it can form the basis for quantitative risk assessment.

hands, leading to discomfort or injury such as grazed knuckles. Also wheelchair access is often placed at the back of a building rather than the main entrance used by able-bodied individuals, reinforcing a sense of exclusion. Toilets designed to provide space to enable a transfer from either the left or right side may exclude those with unilateral impairments.

Universal Design Principles

Inclusive design attempts to deal proactively with capability–demand mismatches by aiming to design equipment, tasks and environments to make them usable by as many people as possible. Universal design attempts to take this a step further, trying to make them usable by *all*. Given the huge range of human capabilities, and the fact that competing goals need to be balanced, this is unlikely to be possible. However, the principles of universal design may well be useful for you to consider when assessing equipment, tasks and environments. It is also worth considering that the same principles should apply to education and training – such materials also need to be accessible and usable, and this is particularly important given how much of education and training in health and social care is now delivered remotely, without direct support for navigating electronic packages.

There are seven principles of universal design (Connell et al., 1997) (Figure 4.4):

1. Equitable use: Can anyone use it?
2. Flexibility in use: Is there more than one way to use it?
3. Simple and intuitive use: When we consider this, in HF/E parlance, we are talking about 'affordances' and 'constraints'. Affordances are perceived and actual properties of a piece of equipment that give clues to how you should operate it. How many times have you stood in front of unfamiliar equipment and thought 'But what do I *do*?' Affordances are often described as 'suggesting the range of possibilities'. Similarly, 'constraints' limit these alternatives – if there were too many different options, then the device would still be difficult to use.
4. Perceptible information: Is it easy to discern relevant information? How is this information presented? Is it visual, aural or tactile? Does it present information in more than one mode (think about user capabilities)? Does the equipment provide feedback so you know that it is responding to an input you have made?
5. Tolerance for (recoverable) error: If you make a mistake, is there feedback that helps you recognise you've made a mistake, and can you undo that mistake?
6. Low physical effort: Think of motor skills, strength and so on, as well as how long you would be expected to use the equipment or carry out the task.
7. Size and space for approach and use: This is especially important in (a) the design of brand-new purpose-built facilities, but also (b) retrofitting of old buildings. When considering what equipment will be used and what tasks will be carried out in a particular space, it is important to think about the people that will be using that space. You also have to consider users who may have assistive technologies, such as wheelchairs, and this will require the allocation of much more space. The safety of the environment may also be relevant, for example, a primary care consulting room could be arranged to ensure an easy exit for clinicians to mitigate the risk to a sole practitioner dealing with a confrontational or aggressive consultation.

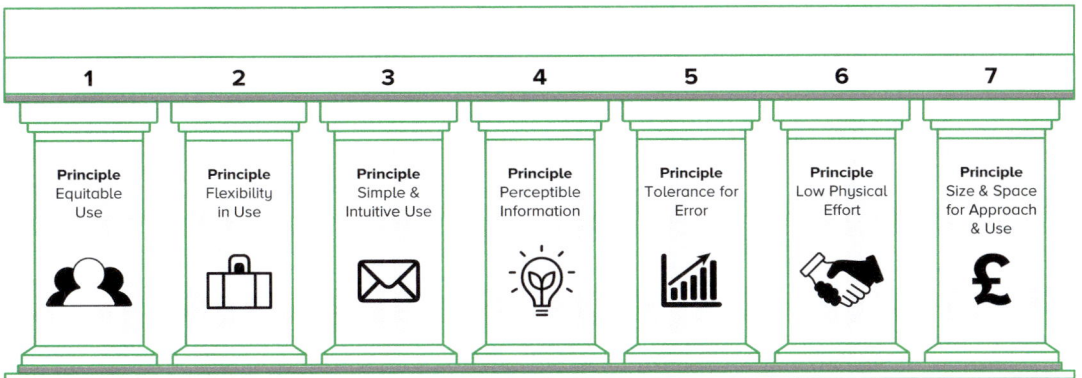

FIGURE 4.4 The Seven Principles of Universal Design.
Source: Based on Connell et al., 1997.

Having considered task and equipment demands and user capability, it is possible to gain some insight into the proportion of users with certain impairments who may be unable to use the product. The Inclusive Design Toolkit (Cambridge Engineering Design Centre, 2015), developed by the Engineering Design Centre at Cambridge University, includes an 'exclusion calculator', which allows a designer or evaluator to predict exclusion based on six key capabilities (vision, hearing, cognitive, locomotion, reach and dexterity). The 'lite' version is free to use, but there are 'paid for' options with more features. A quick look at the calculator, just considering visual capability, suggests that having to read text the size of the print in a newspaper article excludes 4.6% of the population aged between 16 and 64. However, if we change that age range to 65–74, then 10.6% will be excluded. That is interesting when you think of an ageing workforce struggling to interact with increasingly wordy procedures.

Considering capability–demand theory can support an organisational proactive safety strategy, to avoid introducing risks that may be created if the design of equipment is not fit for the intended work environment, population of users or recognised limitations associated with human performance.

Practical Methods for Capturing User Experience and Requirements

Many sectors embed user engagement as part of procurement practice. A 'whole lifecycle' approach is taken, aiming to capture the wider picture, including understanding the skills and competencies required by users and the training needs that this will generate. Such processes are not normally found within health and social care. Without such activity, we don't have the knowledge base from which to make sensible decisions around tasks, processes and equipment design to support user performance. Two methods that may be useful for you to help begin to build your local knowledge base include mapping workshops and personas.

Mapping Workshops

Mapping workshops are useful if you have a particular problem you need to explore. Buckle et al. (2006) describe an application to medication labelling and packaging.

They identified likely stakeholders and divided these into groups, including primary and secondary care deliverers, supply chain stakeholders and patient support groups. Each group attended a separate workshop, where facilitated discussion was used to unpick the user experience in more detail. These discussions can be recorded and then treated as qualitative data, which can be processed further through thematic analysis. The use of rich pictures is encouraged as a mechanism for directing the discussion. Rich pictures encourage people to try to clarify their thinking around complex and ill-defined problems by drawing a picture. Group rich pictures facilitate the building of a shared model, and the discussion required to come up with this shared output is likely to reveal a great deal of information about the problem.

An example of a rich picture is provided in Figure 4.5. This was created to build a persona for 'Jessie' – an older patient living in Shetland but having to travel to Aberdeen by air for treatment for breast cancer. The project was exploring the challenges of older and disabled people accessing air travel. The images included reflect the fact that Jessie doesn't enjoy travel anymore now that she is old and ill, but that she has good family and wider community support back at home. Managing her health is made additionally challenging by her long-standing diabetes. The wheelchair captures the fact that Jessie feels that the air travel environment renders her disabled, especially after she has undergone medical treatment. The items included are 'evidence-based' (from literature and interview with patients undergoing similar experiences).

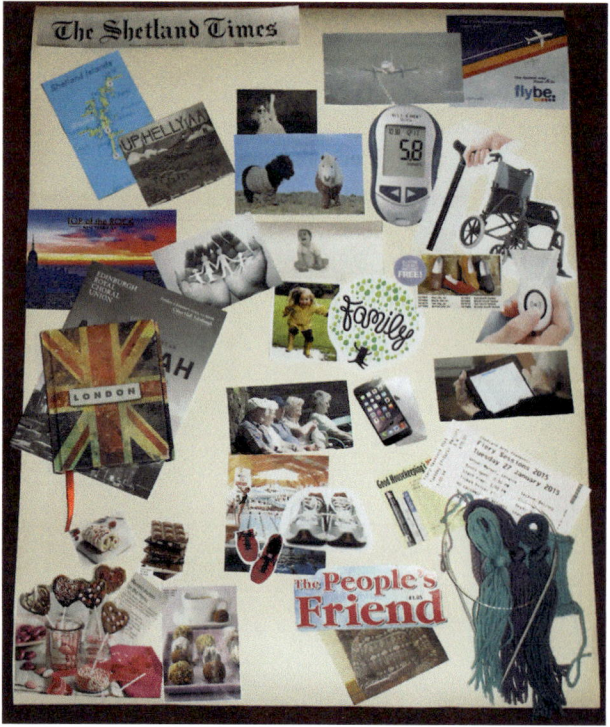

FIGURE 4.5 A 'rich picture'.

Source: © Helen Vosper.

Chapter 4   The People

Personas

Personas help analysts to view a service from the user's perspective and to communicate user needs to other stakeholders (Miaskiewicz, 2011). They are fictitious descriptions of different user types and can be considered a synthesis of multiple users sharing similar goals and behaviours (Marshall et al., 2015). Descriptions of personas include demographic data, motivations, goals, capabilities, skills and attitudes (Clarkson et al., 2015). For example, one such persona is Mary Smith, a 75-year-old former teacher with little IT experience. Mary is left-handed and suffers with failing eyesight. How does this persona inform the design of a self-check-in hospital admission system?

Multiple personas are usually developed to cover the spectrum of user capability. If there is an archetypal user, it makes sense to include this, but often a better analysis can be obtained by considering the case of the 'boundary user', which means someone who can use the equipment or perform the task without help, but experiences difficulty. Personas can be data- or assumption-driven. Data-driven personas are likely to give the best outcome. Data can be drawn from focus groups, field studies and interviews, and user observation. However, data quoted is often discrete – for example, the number of people with a visual impairment. Impairments often occur together, and multi-variate correlation data is difficult to obtain and interpret.

With assumption-driven personas there is a danger of stereotyping, with the developed persona displaying characteristics that the creator believes to be representative. For all personas, developing a rounded character is considered important, but the more specific the characterisation, the smaller the proportion of the total user population it represents. Personas may be particularly useful for improving the user experience for health technology (Holden et al., 2017).

So far we have discussed people within the system as individuals, but another important aspect that affects overall system performance is how effectively individuals are able to work together and communicate with each other as part of teams. This aspect of system performance is often grouped together under the heading 'non-technical skills', and this will be covered in the next chapter (Chapter 5).

Chapter Summary

In this chapter you learnt about the need to reconcile the requirements of tasks, equipment and environment to the capability of the user. The chapter has prompted you to understand the people in the system and the potential mismatch between human capabilities and the expectations or contexts they are required to work in or experience. The information described in this chapter will enable you to start to critically identify or consider performance-influencing factors and user requirements when designing or evaluating work and proactively procuring equipment to accommodate the people in the system. This approach can improve the quality of incident investigations, the development of safety improvements and, more broadly, the design of work and procurement of equipment.

CIEHF HF/E Competencies

Use of a human-centred approach to the design and development of systems
- Understands the role and application of HF/E principles in optimising system performance and well-being across all ages and capabilities.
- Demonstrates ability to enhance health, safety, comfort, quality of life, attitudes, motivation, usability, effectiveness and efficiency.
- Understands the theoretical and practice bases for HF/E relating to design and development of systems.

Focus on how other system components and performance-influencing factors affect people
- Demonstrates use of HF/E theories, methods and tools for analysis of systems (including process), tasks, workload (physical and mental) including mental models, communication and anthropometry.

Human characteristics, capabilities and limitations
- Understands the theoretical and practice bases for HF/E relating to physical capabilities and limitations.
- Understands the influence of such factors as a person's body size, skill, cognitive abilities, age, sensory capacity, general health and experience.
- Determines the match and the interaction between human characteristics, abilities, capacities and motivations, and the system(s), organisation, planned or existing environment, products used, equipment, work systems, machines and tasks.
- Recognises psychological characteristics and responses and how these affect health, human performance, attitudes, perception, stress, human reliability and error.

References

Association of Anaesthetists. 2023. *Fight fatigue resources*. https://anaesthetists.org/Home/Wellbeing-support/Fatigue/-Fight-Fatigue-download-our-information-packs

Buckle, P., Clarkson, P.J., Coleman, R., et al. 2006. Patient safety, systems design and ergonomics. *Applied Ergonomics*, 37(4), 491–500.

Cambridge Engineering Design Centre. 2015. *Exclusion Calculator Lite v2.1. Calc.* inclusivedesigntoolkit.com. https://calc.inclusivedesigntoolkit.com/

Carayon, P., Wetterneck, T.B., Rivera-Rodriguez, A.J., et al. 2014. Human factors systems approach to healthcare quality and patient safety. *Applied Ergonomics*, 45(1), 14–25.

Charles, R. L. & Nixon, J. 2019. Measuring mental workload using physiological measures: A systematic review. *Applied Ergonomics*, 74, 221–232.

Chartered Institute of Ergonomics and Human Factors. 2023. *How to carry out human factors assessments of critical tasks: Guidance for COMAH establishments*. https://ergonomics.org.uk/resource/comah-guidance.html

Clarkson, P. J., Waller, S. & Cardoso, C. 2015. Approaches to estimating user exclusion. *Applied Ergonomics*, 46, 304–310.

Connell, B. R., Jones M.L, Mace, R. L., et al. 1997. The *Principles of Universal Design*, Version 2.0, Raleigh, N.C.: Center for Universal Design, North Carolina State University.

Dawson, D. & McCulloch, K. 2005. Managing fatigue: It's about sleep. *Sleep Medicine*, 9, 365–380.

Folkard, S., & Lombardi, D. A. 2004. Toward a "Risk Index" to Assess Work Schedules. *Chronobiology International*, 21(6), 1063–1072.

Gurubhagavatula, I., Barger, L., Barnes, C., et al. 2021. Guiding principles for determining work shift duration and addressing the effects of work shift duration on performance, safety, and health: Guidance from the American Academy of Sleep Medicine and the Sleep Research Society. *Sleep*, 17(11), 2283–2306.

Hart, S.G. & Staveland, L. E. 1988. Development of NASA-TLX (Task Load Index): Results of empirical and theoretical research. In: Hancock, P. A. & Meshkati, N. (eds.), *Human mental workload*. Elsevier Science, pp. 139–183.

Hart, S. G. 2006 NASA-Task Load Index (NASA-TLX): 20 years later. Paper presented at the Human Factors and Ergonomics Society (HFES) 50th annual meeting, San Francisco, CA.

Health and Safety Executive. (n.d.) *Work-related stress and how to manage it*. https://www.hse.gov.uk/stress/overview.htm

Holden, R. J., Kulanthaivel, A., Purkayastha, S., et al. 2017. Know thy eHealth user: Development of biopsychosocial personas from a study of older adults with heart failure. *International Journal of Medical Informatics*, 108, 158–167.

Hoonakker, P., Carayon, P., Gurses, A. P., et al. 2011. Measuring workload of ICU nurses with a questionnaire survey: The NASA Task Load Index (TLX). *IIE Transactions on Healthcare Systems Engineering*, 1(2), 131–143.

HSSIB. 2024. *Fatigue risk in healthcare and its impact on patient safety*. https://www.hssib.org.uk/patient-safety-investigations/fatigue-risk-in-healthcare-and-its-impact-on-patient-safety/

Huggins, A., & Claudio, D. 2018. A performance comparison between the subjective workload analysis technique and the NASA-TLX in a healthcare setting. *IISE Transactions on Healthcare Systems Engineering*, 8(1), 59–71. https://doi.org/10.1080/24725579.2017.1418765

Kayser, K. C., Puig, V. A. & Estepp, J. R. 2022. Predicting and mitigating fatigue effects due to sleep deprivation: A review. *Frontiers in Neuroscience*. 16, 930280.

Marshall, R., Cook, S., Mitchell, V., et al. 2015. Design and evaluation: End users, user data sets and personas. *Applied Ergonomics*, 46, 311–317.

Miaskiewicz, T. 2011. Personas and user-centred design: How can personas benefit product design processes? *Design Studies*, 32, 417–430.

Pheasant, S. & Haslegrave, C.M. 2006. *Bodyspace: Anthropometry, Ergonomics and the Design of Work*. CRC Press.

Pickup, L., Wilson, J. R., Norris, B., et al. 2005. The Integrated Workload Scale (IWS): A new self report tool to assess railway signaller workload. *Applied Ergonomics*, 36, 681–693.

Reid, G. B. & Nygren, T. E. 1988. The subjective workload assessment technique: A scaling procedure for measuring mental workload. In: Hancock, A. & Meshkati, N. (eds.), *Human mental workload*. Elsevier Science, pp. 185–218.

Salminen, S. 2010. Shift work and extended working hours as risk factors for occupational injury. *The Ergonomics Open Journal*, 3, 14–18.

Tully, P.A., McGagh, B., Ng, D., et al. 2021. Improving the WHO Surgical Safety Checklist sign-out. *BJS Open*, 5(3), zrab028.

Ward, J., Buckle, P. & Clarkson, P. J. 2010. Designing packaging to support the safe use of medicines at home. *Applied Ergonomics*, 41, 682–694.

West, M. A. 2021. *Compassionate leadership sustaining wisdom, humanity and presence in health and social care*. Swirling Leaf Press.

Williamson, A. & Feyer, A. 2000. Sleep deprivation produces impairments in cognitive and motor performance equivalent to legally prescribed levels of alcohol intoxication. *Occupational and Environmental Medicine*, 57, 649–655.

Young, M. S., Brookhuis, K. A., Wickens, C.D., et al. 2014. State of science: Mental workload in ergonomics. *Ergonomics*, 139, 1–17.

CHAPTER 5
Teamwork and Non-Technical Skills

Chapter Objectives and Learning Outcomes

- To understand why teamwork and cognitive skills are important for performance, safety and well-being.
- Present representative approaches to understanding and improving teamwork.
- Discuss different approaches to understanding cognition within work contexts.
- Consider approaches for intervention and reflect on some of the challenges of using this approach for improvement.

Introduction: Understanding the Social, Cognitive and Personal Skills that Enable People to Perform Tasks in the Work Environment

Interactions between people are a prerequisite of safe, efficient and effective care delivery. Team members support each other, watch out for each other, share workload, perform complementary tasks, provide different perspectives and expertise, and make decisions together. Many teams in health and social care are extremely diverse in experience – from novice to 'old hand' – expertise, training, perspective and culture. Even though teamwork and communication are often seen as a source of harm, they are also a source of strength; indeed, the implication of poor teamwork and communication in patient harm events is a demonstration of how reliant we are on teams. There has been a growing science and practical knowledge about what good teamwork looks like, how it can be developed through training, and the contextual factors that enhance, limit, or define the team requirements for success in the first place.

Teamwork and cognition are broad areas with many different schools of thought. Dedicated books provide comprehensive overviews; for example, *Safety at the sharp end: A guide to non-technical skills* considers topics such as situation awareness, decision making, communication, teamwork and leadership (Flin and O'Connor, 2017). However, in line with systems thinking, introduced in Chapter 1, in this chapter we will take a different approach and explore teamwork as an emergent outcome of interactions of the elements of the work system, rather than as a property that resides exclusively within individuals. Table 5.1 outlines key systems-thinking principles that can help understand team performance.

We will discuss teamwork principles in general, with a focus on three teamwork frameworks. Next, we review the concept of cognition, also with a focus on three models. Finally, we describe implementation of training and other improvement methods, and, given how popular these approaches have been within patient safety, offer some words of caution.

TABLE 5.1 Systems-thinking principles for understanding team performance

Team performance emerges from system design.	Team performance should be understood as emerging from system design, which enables good team performance. This offers a more fruitful perspective rather than regarding team performance as the result of a set of teamworking behaviours, which are somehow unconnected to the wider system. The focus should, therefore, be on understanding and designing interactions between, for example, people and the tools they use, the spaces within which people work, as well as the cultures within an organisation.
The physical environment can have a significant influence on team performance.	An example of the systems perspective is consideration of how the physical environment impacts team performance. Co-creation and maintenance of a shared vision is facilitated by people being in the same physical space rather than in separate spaces (for example, 'nurses' station' and 'doctor's office').
	Effective environmental layout of workspaces can also provide opportunities for communication and can reduce the need for potentially unnecessary communication, which otherwise could be perceived as a nuisance and detrimental to teamwork. For example, having a clear line of sight to a piece of information or equipment such that the need for interrupting a colleague and having to ask for information is reduced.
The organisation of work should be designed with the multi-disciplinary team in mind rather than along professional boundaries.	Work activities are frequently still designed according to professional boundaries, for example, grand rounds tend to involve only doctors because nurses cannot leave their wards.
	The organisation of work should consider the needs of multi-disciplinary working, and this should be designed into work activities. Examples might include activities that are designed into daily structures, such as multi-professional huddles and multi-professional simulations. Existing task design can be siloed and separated (for example, nurse tasks, doctor tasks), and this can cause divisions.

External and organisational pressures challenge effective team performance.	Embracing challenges and pressures, for example in competitive sports, can be highly motivating. However, pressures in healthcare are often operational and manifest themselves in staff and resource shortages over prolonged periods of time. This can have the opposite effect, that is, it can be highly frustrating, and it can lead to stress, fatigue and staff burnout, especially if the individual has a lack of control over the situation. This can have significantly detrimental effects on overall team performance.
The culture in healthcare is changing, but it can still undermine effective team performance.	There is a push in healthcare for systems thinking and a culture that does not apportion blame to individuals, but which supports and engages compassionately with those affected by incidents. However, the culture across a health system, such as the NHS, is not uniform, and in many teams and organisations there persists a blame culture, which can lead to dysfunctional team performance.

Teamwork in Health and Social Care

A team is usually described as two or more individuals who (Tannenbaum and Salas, 2020):

- Socially interact
- Possess one or more common goals
- Are brought together to perform organisationally relevant tasks
- Exhibit interdependencies with respect to workflow, goals and outcomes
- Have different roles and responsibilities
- Are together embedded in an encompassing organisational system, with boundaries and linkages to the broader system context and task environment.

Teams are required for most aspects of health and social care, including diagnosis and treatment. Different professionals with diverse expertise, such as doctors, nurses and specialists, collaborate to evaluate a patient's condition and develop a comprehensive treatment plan. Teams play a crucial role in planning and ongoing evaluation. They regularly reassess the patient's progress and adjust the treatment plan accordingly to ensure optimal outcomes. This collaborative approach improves the overall quality of care provided. Team activities also serve as instructive and informative opportunities. Health and social care professionals engage in teaching and learning activities to enhance their knowledge and skills. They discuss evidence-based practices, share experiences, and update each other with the latest research findings. This continuous learning improves the overall competence of the team and ultimately benefits patients and service users. Assigning more experienced staff members to challenging patients or service users ensures that complex cases receive the specialised attention they require.

Team activities can occur synchronously or asynchronously. Synchronous activities involve face-to-face meetings, phone calls, or video conferences and telehealth sessions, allowing immediate interaction and real-time decision making. Asynchronous activities, on the other hand, involve communication through text messages, email, pagers, chart records, notes, stickers or annotations. These methods enable communication over extended periods, allowing for flexibility in exchanging information. Building strong relationships and effective communication among team members create a positive work environment. This, in turn, enhances collaboration and promotes better care. It is important to note that teams are not limited to a single group. In reality, individuals are members of multiple teams that form and interact based on the needs of individual patients and service users. Care delivery teams also rely on a large number of intersecting support teams, such as laboratory, porters, environmental services, security, logistics, maintenance and administration teams.

While the ultimate goal of these teams is always to deliver safe and effective care for patients or service users, the means by which this is achieved, and the necessary trade-offs involved, can differ among team members. Teams are comprised of individuals with shared goals, performing relevant tasks within an organisational system. Team members usually have a wide array of expertise and backgrounds, resulting in a rich tapestry of perspectives, opinions, approaches, languages, motivations and world views. This diversity serves as both a source of strength and a potential weakness. On one hand, it allows for the availability of different perspectives on potential options and treatments, but on the other hand, it can give rise to disagreements and conflicts due to differing perspectives on the best course of action. These conflicts should not be viewed as inherently negative. Rather, they highlight the existence of multiple potential options in any given situation. To ensure fruitful collaboration, it is crucial for team members to possess not only task-specific skills, but also effective teamwork, co-ordination and communication skills. The ability to speak the same 'language' in terms of teamwork enables cohesion and enhances the overall effectiveness of the team.

Teamwork and communication play a significant role in delivering safe and high-quality care. Unfortunately, these skills are not always emphasised or formally taught, especially in healthcare education. As a result, healthcare professionals may be lacking in this aspect, hindering their ability to work cohesively as a team.

One common issue that hinders effective teamwork is the reluctance to 'speak up' about problems. Hierarchical tensions within healthcare organisations can create a culture where lower-ranked team members hesitate to voice their concerns or suggestions. This lack of open communication can compromise patient safety. Another challenge arises during handovers or transitions of care, where critical information can get lost, leading to errors or omissions in patient management. This breakdown in communication can have serious consequences, as essential details may 'fall between the cracks', leaving team members uninformed.

Initiatives that focus on enhancing teamwork and communication abilities have demonstrated considerable value in improving safety, efficiency and patient outcomes. Teamwork improvement interventions often focus on training to change behaviours. Team-based learning and simulation allow for specific scenarios to be practised and reinforced, but caution must be exercised as training can be costly and may not address broader systemic factors. Teamwork is not just about individual and collective skills but should also consider the broader context in which it occurs. Taking a 'systems approach' in health and social care allows us to understand how various factors interact to foster the teamwork that drives safe and effective care. Other approaches, such as checklists, structured briefings, and debriefings, can support team processes and decision making. Combining skills training with systematic support is more likely to be effective.

The Seven Cs Model

One of the most rigorously researched frameworks for understanding teamwork across application contexts is the 'Seven Cs' model established by Salas at al. over many years (Tannenbaum and Salas, 2020). This research started in military applications and has been applied broadly across many different industries, as well as in healthcare. The Seven Cs are:

1. Capability – a successful team requires the right mix of people with the right skills.
2. Co-operation – team members have to be willing to work together to achieve a shared goal, rather than just focusing on one personal goal. They have to be willing to give and receive input from others on the team.
3. Co-ordination – teams have to behave in ways that allow the sharing of the goals and tasks, so, for example, understanding that what one member does might affect the other(s).
4. Communication – team members have to exchange information in order to share tasks and understand progress towards a goal. This should be clear, succinct and timely.
5. Cognition – team members need to have a shared understanding of the current situation, the goals, and the tasks, team members and resources required to reach them.
6. Coaching – teams rarely suddenly function well immediately but need to be facilitated by leaders who build trust, set standards, resolve conflicts and act as coaches.
7. Conditions – effective teams need appropriate resources, working environments, organisational support and incentives to function. This is sometimes called 'culture'.

The Seven Cs model is useful because it defines a set of principles that include structural and behavioural components, acknowledging that both the skills of the individuals and the design of the teams and their context are important for effective teamwork. This is valuable to think about within a health and social care context as, alone, behavioural approaches may not be enough. The downside of this model is that it does not offer any specific guidance for any one team. As we will explore, the more specificity in a teamwork approach, the better for application, but the less transferable the learning.

TeamSTEPPS

Perhaps the best recognised collection of teamwork skills in healthcare is the Team Strategies and Tools to Enhance Performance and Patient Safety (TeamSTEPPS) (King et al., 2008). Developed in the mid-2000s as a comprehensive approach to patient safety teamwork challenges, it was derived from prior work in military, aviation and other high-risk industries. It is organised into four themes: leadership, communication, mutual support and situation monitoring. It also includes modules on critical communications protocols, readbacks and checkbacks, handovers and handoffs, briefs, debriefs and huddles, checklists, situation awareness and cross-monitoring, feedback, and approaches for speaking up. However, the abundance of materials can be overwhelming, and as the critical aspects of performance vary between teams, the specific application of TeamSTEPPS principles may differ depending on the context. The generic curriculum does not cater to the unique needs of each team, requiring learners to interpret and apply it themselves. It also needs to be purposefully configured and receive long-term support from departmental and organisational leadership. The materials are downloadable for free, with train-the-trainer courses readily available.

Non-Technical Skills Frameworks

The concept of non-technical skills (NTS) arises from the idea that while there are specialist 'technical' skills required to complete complex tasks (such as knowing a surgical procedure, the instruments and equipment needed, and the specific actions to perform), there are a set of more 'non-technical' skills that are also necessary for success. These are generally considered as teamwork, leadership and social skills, as well as cognitive skills such as decision making and situation awareness. Rather than being just a set of training principles, NTS frameworks usually offer a set of observational templates – behavioural marker systems – that allow the development, evaluation and certification of NTS through the observation of these behaviours as the work is conducted, either in simulation or during real work. In this respect, NTS frameworks and the behavioural marker systems that emerge from them offer very specific guidance with practical benefits for the ongoing development of these skills.

The most popular healthcare teamwork training frameworks have their roots in crew resource management (CRM), which was developed as part of pilot training from the late 1970s. As safety increased in line with the increased engineered reliability of airframes and engines, accidents that appeared to be rooted in 'aircrew operational relationships' emerged. CRM focused on developing these key NTS through training, feedback, simulation and certification. Figure 5.1 shows the model that underpins CRM thinking, with *outcomes* delivered as a result of *processes*, that *transform* the inputs to outputs. If NTS development is to be successful, it needs not just active training of team processes, but also consideration of elements in the wider work system, and as such shares similarities with the SEIPS (Systems Engineering Initiative for Patient Safety) model. CRM has continued to develop since then, although much of what has been applied in healthcare is based on earlier models.

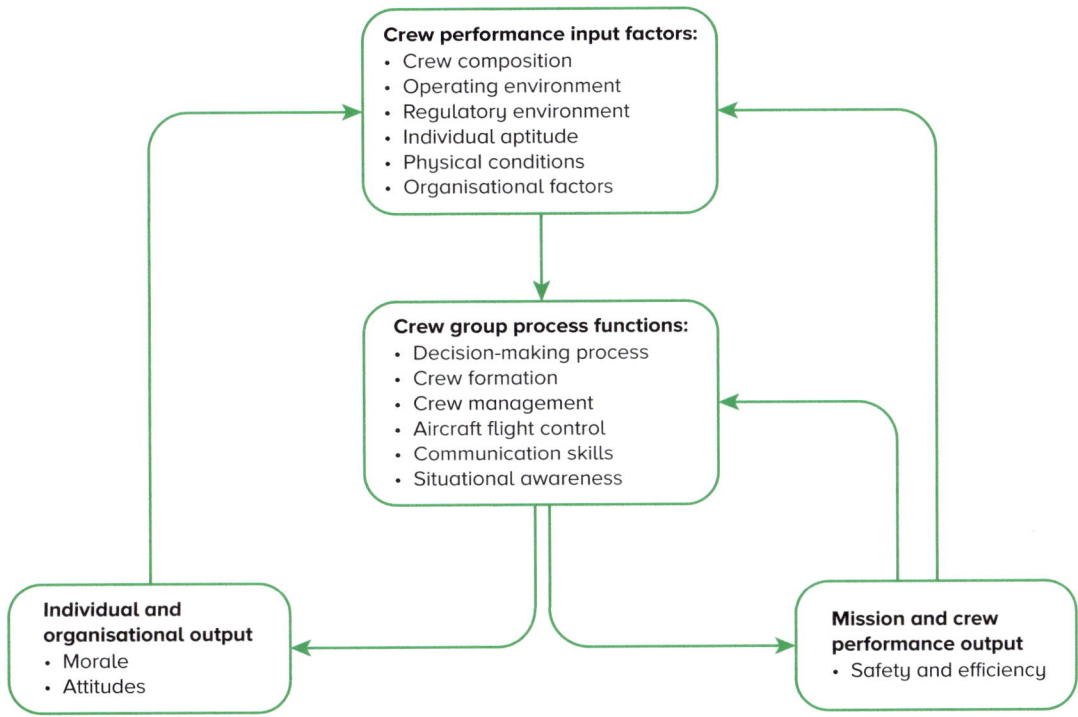

FIGURE 5.1 Input-process-output model.
Source: Based on Helmreich and Foushee, 1993.

Many NTS tools are available for assessing competencies since the first adoption by healthcare of the non-technical skills assessment framework (NOTECHS) (Flin et al., 2003). Many of the tools have been extensively used in operating theatre environments (for surgeons, anaesthetists, anaesthetic nurses, for example), while others have been developed to focus on specific aspects of the NTS 'bundle', such as teamworking. A systematic review by Higham et al. (2019) provides an overview of tools currently used and their contexts.

What comprises effective NTS varies from role to role and within different contexts. As with TeamSTEPPS and the Seven Cs model, there is a trade-off between generalisability and specificity. A more general approach will be able to cover more disciplines or specialties at the expense of the specificity that is needed to guide particular behaviours. Effective NTS in cardiac surgery are particularly dependent upon the sharing of information, tasks and decision making between the surgeon, the anaesthetist and the perfusionist. However, knee replacement surgery depends upon a scrub nurse who knows how the surgical equipment for that brand of prosthetic is used, and a surgeon who is able to use it. The anaesthetist may communicate only briefly with the rest of the team, while a change in the brand of prosthetic can significantly reduce performance and situation awareness. Similarly, there can be different demands for robotic surgery or other surgical technologies. Thus, there is no one right set of behavioural markers, and developing specific guidance for each role can be challenging and time consuming.

Cognition, Situation Awareness, Sense Making and Decision Making

Aligned with these behavioural approaches to teamwork, there has been considerable interest and success across a range of industries for identifying and developing approaches to understanding and improving cognition. In any context, we seek to make sense of the world around us using the information available and the knowledge or experience we have to interpret and recognise familiar patterns to inform the decisions and actions we take. Expertise is reflected in knowing which information sources to check and noticing what is important, understanding what the cues that you notice are telling you about the world around you, and where this is currently leading the situation (and thus the actions required of you to get to where you want to be). Experts often have a remarkable capacity to 'think ahead' to give them the best chance of achieving their goals and of avoiding an accident. The most effective form of safe practice is avoiding risky situations altogether by anticipating and navigating away from them. It is also said that the first sign of something going wrong is to be unable to predict what is likely to happen. Seeking to understand why decisions made sense, and seeking to facilitate a work system to support better decision making, requires insight into the context, the person and human cognition. Although the consideration of human perception and cognition is far too broad a topic to address here, even within HF/E practice, let alone in the broader experimental psychology or cognitive science domains, we have chosen to focus on three well-used frameworks.

Possibly the most frequently used – and consequently the most frequently misapplied – approach to cognition within safety is the concept of 'situation awareness' (SA). SA theory describes three levels of awareness about a task or a constantly changing situation that contribute to performance (Endsley, 1995). Level 1 SA, 'Noticing', describes how, in order to begin to understand the world around us, we first have to detect an important piece of information within the environment. Level 2 SA, 'Understanding', relates to the meaning that is applied to the information that you have noticed. It is one thing to note an increase in blood pressure, but another to know what that means for the physiological state of the patient right now. Level 3 SA, 'Projecting', is the highest level of SA and relates to the ability to understand what will be happening in the future, based on your current understanding of the world and how it is changing. Box 5.1 illustrates the concept of situation awareness using a driving task and clinical tasks on a ward.

The advantage of SA is that it is a relatively simple introduction to meta-cognition, that is, thinking about thinking. It has face validity in being easily relatable to all manner of everyday situations, and particularly to high-risk or highly technical activity. However, the generically applicable, easy initial comprehensibility, and lack of specificity of SA has meant that it is frequently cited as a cause in incident investigations. Essentially, as something bad happened, investigators are tempted to conclude that it must have involved a loss of SA, with the assumption being that this would not have happened if SA had been sufficient. As well as being simply an artefact of hindsight bias, when combined with a lack of consideration as to where

Chapter 5 Teamwork and Non-Technical Skills

BOX 5.1 Examples of situation awareness in driving and clinical tasks

Situation awareness in daily driving

Imagine you are driving down the motorway in the slow lane. You notice an exit coming up, which means you understand and rightly predict that there will also be a slip road onto the motorway. You scan ahead to the slip road and notice that there is a car travelling down it, intending to come onto the motorway. You already understand that this car will be coming into your lane, and immediately try to predict whether it will arrive on the motorway before, after, or at the same time that you reach the point where it will join. Based on your speed and the speed you observe of the other vehicle, you predict that there is a chance of collision if things stay as they are. Action is necessary, either to speed up, slow down, or change to a different lane. You check your rear-view mirror and blind spot, and notice that there is a van next to you, which means that you cannot change to the middle lane right now, but if you slow down a little, in a moment the van will be past. This means you can move into the middle lane in plenty of time to avoid a collision. As you slow down, you notice that the car on the slip road has been accelerating, which means that you now predict it will join the motorway well before you, and thus there is no longer a danger. You continue to observe the relative speed of the vehicles close to you as you continue on your way.

Situation awareness in clinical tasks on a ward

It is 7:30pm on a busy ward, and nurse Jeremy is looking after three patients: Rose, Bob and Jane. Rose can't make it to the bathroom safely on her own, and it's been several hours since she went, so nurse Jeremy knows he needs to check in on her. Meanwhile, Bob's wife and kids have just arrived and are eager to see him and get an update on his progress. Finally, Jane needs a line changing, and Jeremy has just noticed that Megan, the rounding registrar, has arrived on the ward and might be available to do that. Recognising that he does not want Rose to try to get up on her own, as falls are a high risk, and that Bob's family will be able to wait a minute or two, Jeremy first asks Megan to see to Jane's line, then asks Bob's family to wait for just a minute while he goes to check on Rose. Rose says she's okay for now but might be ready soon, so Jeremy invites Bob's family into his room, and they speak for a few minutes. Once their questions are answered, Jeremy checks with Megan that the line has been changed and that everything looks good with Jane, then goes back to Rose's room and takes her to the bathroom.

SA is derived from, what it might consist of within a given context, whether that was knowable, or the task conditions under which it might degrade, 'loss of SA' becomes a surrogate for blame.

More recently, the Distributed Situation Awareness (DSA) model emphasises the systems perspective on SA (Stanton et al., 2006). According to the DSA model, SA is distributed around the sociotechnical system, and is built through interactions between agents, both human (for example, clinicians) and even non-human (for example, AI systems). Critically, the SA required for successful performance is not held by any one agent alone, and different agents have different views on the same situation, which need to be compatible. SA is developed and updated dynamically through SA transactions. These exchanges can be human-to-human, human-to-non-human, and non-human-to-non-human (for example, interaction between a monitoring device, such as an ECG, and the AI). For instance, human agents transact with other human agents via communications and non-verbal signals. Technological agents transact with human agents through displays, alarms and warnings, text-based communications, signs, symbols and other aspects relating to their state. Human agents transact with technological agents through data input, and technological agents transact with each other through data transfer and communication protocols. How SA is exchanged between people and AI, and between AI and other systems, is thus a critical design consideration. In turn, this requires an understanding of the SA requirements of all components of the clinical system.

The example provided in Box 5.2 captures themes recognised within the field of maternity. This would refocus us to reflect on the *equipment* and *technology* or

BOX 5.2 Situation awareness arising from interactions of elements of the work system in a maternity context

> Maternity staff have to process different types of information in the context of uncertainty and emerging signs and symptoms indicating different stages of labour. The risks associated with labour make it essential for staff to complete time-critical and regular assessments of different clinical signs and emerging situations. The information they rely upon may stem from a woman calling in via the telephone and describing different symptoms; staff are required to triage based on this communication and estimate the urgency with which admission is required. The experience of staff answering the call, access to any relevant medical history or record of the number of previous calls made and the use of a shared language may all influence the assessment and outcome. This process is safety critical, as it forms the gateway to the opportunity for a more detailed assessment and gathering of relevant information through physical observations and examination.
>
> Once admitted into a healthcare setting, there are different tools used to establish the health of and risk to the baby and mother. The availability of tools to measure the baby's heart rate is heavily relied upon, but may differ depending upon the maternity setting. The documentation of observations and critical metrics, such as heart rate of both baby and mother, may be dependent upon organisational pressures and demand on services, usability of equipment and the familiarity of staff with specific equipment. As different team members are required to assist or provide opinions, they may have differing levels and quality of information in this frequently fast-moving context. The equipment relied upon to interpret the heart rate of the baby varies in its usability and reliability, hence the assessment of this situation can only be as good as the information available to the clinician.

interface design. Consideration should be given to the usability of the technology and its ability to provide an effective representation of all necessary information. Furthermore, we would also want to understand how the system can alert the user to a change in status of the system and the reliability and quality in the transfer of information. These factors will all influence the user's trust and ability to interpret and obtain an accurate mental model of any emerging situation. How does the *environment* influence the ability to obtain and access information or *people* to ensure an accurate picture of events? How does the *organisation* arrange work, people or teams and the physical space or equipment they work with? Reflecting on the elements of the system offers a tangible view on why (or why not) staff may (or may not) be able to notice, understand and predict emerging situations. This shifts the emphasis back to the work system to enable SA rather than it being seen as a property of an individual and something to be 'lost'. Thus, SA is not just a property residing in the mind of the individual, but also of the system to allow SA to form and be maintained.

Other Decision-Making Models

The reality of decision making in health and social care is one where information is often incomplete, delayed and not everything can be predicted. This complex and dynamic working environment requires acceptance that adjustments are required as information materialises, or sense is made of a situation. Trade-offs are likely as goals shift or risks become more or less relevant to achieving the goals of patient safety, service efficiency and optimal professional performance. To promote a just culture, this perspective needs to be considered when retrospectively looking at an unintended outcome (incident reviews), as well as considering how to design future work systems and procedures.

The recognition-primed decision (RPD) model explains how situation assessment and sense-making processes assist in evaluating options through mental simulation or recognising familiar patterns. Real-world decision making is a product of the knowledge held by staff and the context or environment, which may or may not support how information 'cues' are delivered, recognised and received (Kahneman and Klein, 2009; Klein, 2008. Real-world decision making is recognised as occurring in 'messy' contexts, where uncertainty is common, and staff must make decisions informed by their knowledge and experience to accommodate the uncertainty created by missing or ambiguous information amid other organisational pressures and time-pressured environments (Flach et al., 2017).

'Distributed cognition' (DC) contends that information is stored, acted upon and exchanged across individuals, technologies, cultures and other artefacts, and it is this distribution that leads to effective understanding and decision making in complex systems. In the seminal work 'How a cockpit remembers its speeds', Edwin Hutchins (1995) illustrates how outcomes are not the consequence of the information processing of individuals alone, pointing out that a successful flight relies on two pilots interacting with one another and with a variety of technologies. His examples demonstrate how the properties of such a distributed system can differ from the cognitive properties of the individual humans within them. So, poorly functioning technologies might lead two expert pilots to make what appear to be cognitive or communication errors, but focusing only on the error (or, indeed, 'SA' of the pilots) would be thoroughly misleading. The Distributed Cognition for Teamwork (DiCoT) framework is a way of structuring DC analysis, which has proved successful in the healthcare domain. DiCoT subdivides the analysis into different models: (i) information flow model; (ii) physical model; (iii) artefact model; (iv) social model; (v) evolutionary model. DiCoT thus addresses the multi-dimensionality of patient safety issues and is especially useful for understanding how the environment supports cognition. An example outlining the application of this framework is illustrated by Blandford and Furniss (2005).

Thus, rather than there being only one right way to explore cognition and decision making, the varied ways in which we have to understand the world gives us the opportunity to apply multiple lenses to any health and social care context. There will be more and less appropriate approaches for a given goal, but it's nearly always useful to apply a few different perspectives, as this will almost always provide new ways to think about a given situation or problem.

Delivery

When planning a teamwork improvement intervention, it is worth thinking about some of the stages to work through:

- Initial exploration – understand the context in which teams are working, including member mix and availability, organisational support, shared goals and the working environment.
- Training needs – establish the improvement that you want to achieve through training. Improvements may also be achieved or may need to be supported through structural changes.
- Delivery – through laboratory simulation, in-situ simulation or classroom teaching. This will depend on the training demands and availability of resources. Generally speaking, a combination of classroom and simulation is likely to be more effective than either alone.
- Transference – thinking about how to encourage adoption of the desired behaviours or traits following the training can help transfer that learning to habit. In-situ coaching or weekly follow-up discussions, for example, can help with transference.
- Sustainability – the skills and behaviours that you have established will eventually fade, either because the teams drift back to their prior way of doing things, or the work context changes to meet different demands and priorities, or simply through staff turnover. To realise continued benefits of the initial investment, refresher training, complementary training, training needs reviews and induction training for new members can be provided.

Words of Caution

The popularity of teamwork training as an intervention has led to several misconceptions and ineffective approaches. While aspects of teamwork, especially the NTS and CRM approaches, may sometimes be referred to as 'human factors', as you will see from the structure and content of this book, this in no way represents HF/E as a discipline. Indeed, a focus only on behavioural change is not really systems thinking, and there is a deeper concern that behavioural approaches ignore wider systems issues that affect teamwork and situation awareness. Communication and teamworking might be poor not because of limitations of the individuals involved, but because the system-of-work is not well designed to support effective communication. If this is the case, then no amount of teamwork or NTS training will solve the problem. Improving teamwork is never just about telling someone through a set of slides that they should do something differently. Indeed, training is usually recognised as being among the least effective ways to improve performance and safety. Without careful consideration of how teamwork and behaviours emerge from systems properties, teamwork and NTS training represent an unwelcome return to a 'blame and retrain' approach.

Even if specific behaviours can be identified, and a means to improvement carefully developed, there are still many challenges. People cannot be trained if they are not willing to be trained, and there remains considerable resistance to what are perceived as 'soft skills' by many clinicians. Resistance to teamwork training can also be understandable if the trainees feel that other aspects of the work organisation are ignored, and it can feel like members are being blamed for deeper systemic threats to safety or performance that the training does not address. Behaviour is heavily influenced by context, and in the face of, say, 20 years of otherwise successful practice, it can be difficult to change familiar habits, even if the intention is aligned. Together, this means that the success of any teamwork intervention can be brittle in the face of other organisational and professional influences. While training may initially be an attractive and straightforward approach to improving performance and safety, the work that needs to go into understanding the demands, context and skills necessary, working with the team members to establish the value of and motivation for the change, and the necessary short-term and long-term follow-up mean that this work is neither inexpensive nor easy, and even then it is still unlikely to lead to the exact changes that are intended.

SA has been particularly misunderstood and loosely applied. First, it is a folk model – that is, it can mean different things to different people, so it is not one thing, or even one theory, but a collection of related ideas, which are changed to fit a given situation. Second, as SA can apply at multiple cognitive levels in multiple situations, it is non-specific, and looks very different in very different contexts. Third, it assumes that there is a set of known stimuli through which, with enough cognitive processing and enough expertise, it is possible to arrive at a solution. This may be possible within the original conception of SA as being what was needed to achieve a firing solution during air combat – where the key information is available to the pilot, and the solution can be defined through physics – but this may not suit situations where information is not available, or the goal unclear, or the results of different actions might be strongly mediated by other parameters (such as the unique anatomy and physiology of every patient). Furthermore, it is debatable whether knowing about SA is helpful for obtaining it, so as a teaching tool, it may help to think about thinking and give language to some of those ideas, but it does not help to acquire the context-specific expertise necessary for success. Finally, there is little evidence that SA reflects how our brains actually filter information, so while it might feel 'right', and to a certain extent may reflect some aspects of conscious cognitive processing, it is not sufficient, for example, to describe the non-conscious mechanism by which we will be drawn and respond to specific stimuli or situations. Consequently, 'SA Failure' is rarely a sufficient explanation for an accident and is usually found to be a surrogate for blame. Thus, the strength of SA – that it is easy to understand conceptually and can be applied to virtually any task, clinical or otherwise – is also why it may be of limited value as an explanation for specific behaviours or performance.

Chapter Summary

Effective teamwork and cognition are necessary for the safe and effective delivery of care, so it makes sense to attempt to model, understand and improve these skills, especially given that they have rarely been emphasised in clinical training. This chapter explored teamwork from a systems perspective, that is, as something that arises from and is shaped by the interaction of different elements of the work system, including, for example, the physical environment and organisational factors.

You were introduced to a variety of popular tools and analytical frameworks to understand teamwork and cognition. Though NTS and SA frameworks are particularly popular, the technical challenges of understanding and implementing improvements may not be fully recognised, and there are a number of very difficult limitations to overcome for a successful intervention. Other frameworks may be valuable to consider, and always keeping in mind the influence of the wider system on current and future behaviour is essential for the success of any one teamwork or cognitive intervention.

CIEHF HF/E Competencies

Human capabilities and limitations
- Understands the theoretical and practice bases for HF/E relating to psychological and social capabilities and limitations.

Application of relevant methods, tools and techniques
- Understands theoretical and practice bases for analysis of human interactions.

References

Blandford, A. & Furniss, D. 2005. DiCoT: A methodology for applying distributed cognition to the design of teamworking systems. In: *International workshop on design, specification, and verification of interactive systems*. Springer Berlin Heidelberg, pp. 26–38.
Endsley, M. R. 1995. Toward a theory of situation awareness in a dynamic system. *Human Factors*, 37(1), 32–64.
Flach, J.M., Feufel, M.A., Reynolds, P.L., et al., 2017. Decisionmaking in practice: The dynamics of muddling through. *Applied Ergonomics*, 63, 133–141.
Flin, R., Martin, L., Goeters, K.-M., et al. 2003. Development of the NOTECHS (non-technical skills) system for assessing pilots' CRM skills. *Human Factors and Aerospace Safety*, 3(2), 95–117.

Flin, R. & O'Connor, P. 2017. *Safety at the sharp end: A guide to non-technical skills*. CRC Press.

Helmreich, R. L., & Foushee, H. C. 1993. Why crew resource management? Empirical and theoretical bases of human factors training in aviation. In: E. L. Wiener, B. G. Kanki, & R. L. Helmreich (eds.), *Cockpit resource management*. Academic Press, pp. 3–45.

Higham, H., Greig, P. R., Rutherford, J., et al. 2019. Observer-based tools for nontechnical skills assessment in simulated and real clinical environments in healthcare: A systematic review. *BMJ Quality and Safety*, 28, 672–686.

Hutchins E. 1995. How a cockpit remembers its speed. *Cognitive Science*. 19, 265–288.

Kahneman, D. and Klein, G., 2009. Conditions for intuitive expertise: A failure to disagree. *American psychologist*, 64(6), 515–526.

King, H.B., Battles, J., Baker, D.P., et al. 2008. TeamSTEPPS™: Team Strategies and Tools to Enhance Performance and Patient safety. *Advances in patient safety: New directions and alternative approaches (Vol. 3: Performance and tools)*.

Klein, G., 2008. Naturalistic decision making. *Human factors*, 50(3), 456–460.

Stanton, N. A., Stewart, R., Harris, D., et al. 2006. Distributed situation awareness in dynamic systems: Theoretical development and application of an ergonomics methodology. *Ergonomics*, 49, 1288–1311.

Tannenbaum, S. & Salas, E. 2020. *Teams That Work: The Seven Drivers of Team Effectiveness*. Oxford University Press.

CHAPTER 6

The Environment

Chapter Objectives and Learning Outcomes

- To understand the characteristics of the environment that impact people – service users, patients and staff – and their work and goals.
- To describe the properties of the environment relevant to physical and cognitive performance and well-being – for example, layout, position, noise, temperature, lighting.
- To explore ways in which you might better understand health and social care physical environments as the context of all interactions.
- To have knowledge of basic methods to capture this information and apply it to workplace or safety reviews and incident investigations.

Introduction: Understanding the Context Provided by the Environment and Its Impact on People

The layout, physical environment and the positioning of equipment will all influence the way work is done. While the need for human-centred design of tasks, tools and technology is increasingly being recognised, the impact of the physical environment is easily overlooked and often neglected or added to the 'too hard to change' list. The context that we observe people working within may not have been proactively designed (Figure 6.1), and people have an outstanding capability to adapt and work around obstacles and to problem-solve to achieve tasks even in the most challenging of environments. Hence, the efficiency or safety of tasks may not have been explored, and often little consideration is given to the implications for the physical and psychological well-being of the people using the environment (including service users, patients, staff and visitors).

Typically, healthcare settings are not designed with specific tasks in mind, but rather are inherited by a set of professionals or a clinical department who then fit around the environment. Rarely do staff modify the physical workplace in the context of their work; this may not occur to them, or they may not be empowered to adjust their environments for the purpose of safety, performance or well-being. This chapter will consider the physical context where work is done as influential to performance, safety and well-being of service users, patients and staff.

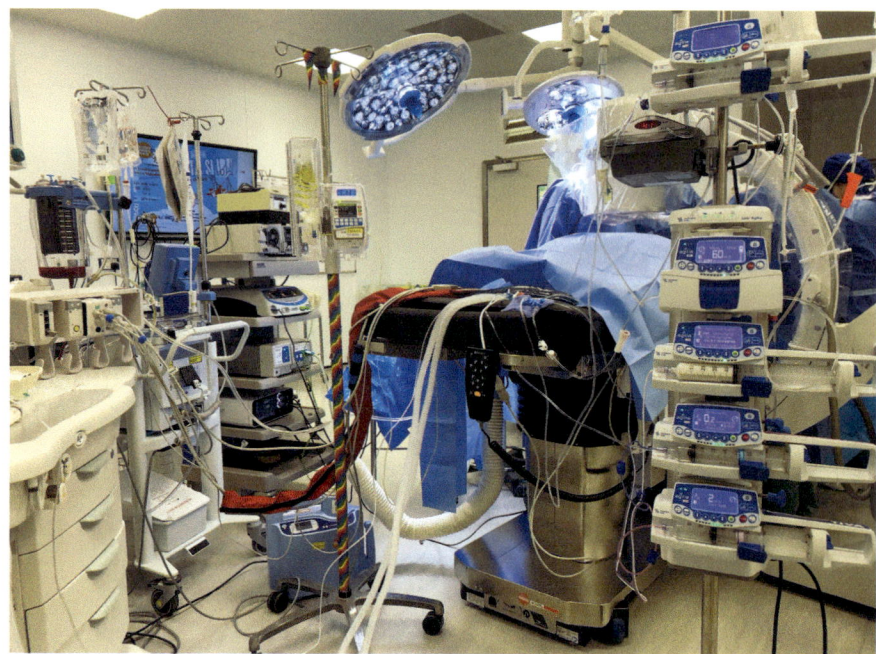

FIGURE 6.1 A typical surgical environment with difficult access to patient, equipment, electrical sockets, as well as trip hazards.

Source: © Danielle Franklin.

This chapter might be of particular use for:

- Proactive identification of workplace hazards
- New design or redesign of environments to support performance, safety and well-being
- Those involved in risk assessing, for example manual handling or falls prevention
- Incident investigation.

Is the Environment Fit for Purpose?

Typically, the term ergonomics is more often used for the science that informs the design and evaluation of physical environments or equipment. The knowledge attributed to the field of ergonomics includes information on physical layouts, noise, lighting and temperature. Each of these areas is recognised as impacting human performance, safety or user experience and has a body of science and regulatory frameworks to inform how we can understand the compatibility between the environment and the person experiencing the environment. As suggested at the start of this book, the terms ergonomics and human factors are interchangeable and do, in fact, cover the same field of science.

The term anthropometry has been described in Chapter 4 (on 'People'). The current chapter will introduce the ways in which anthropometrics can be used to design or evaluate the layout of a physical environment.

Chapter 6 The Environment

Physical Fit Within an Environment

Musculoskeletal injuries are one consequence of a poorly designed physical environment, and they have been within the top two causes of long-term sickness and absence in the UK NHS for many years. At the time of writing approximately 265,000 days were lost in one month due to musculoskeletal problems (NHS Digital, 2022). This has implications for staff well-being and for the retention of staff within the NHS and the availability of staff to meet the needs of patients, not to mention the cost to the NHS. Prevention of physical harm to staff and patients can be influenced through preventative actions to consider how the design of physical workspaces meets the needs of both staff and patients. Here we find not all groups are considered equally when we consider the design of everyday things and environments (see Chapter 10 on 'Equality, Diversity and Inclusion').

A proactive HF/E analysis would consider the tasks and work that are typical to staff and patients within a particular healthcare context. This can reveal how the layout and physical structures may impact on people in different ways and enable work to be completed safely, reliably and with the least effort (Box 6.1).

BOX 6.1 Example – the physical location of a drug cupboard may impact on performance and well-being

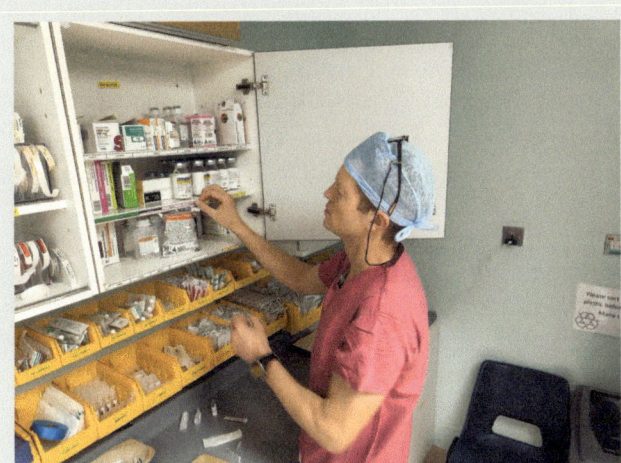
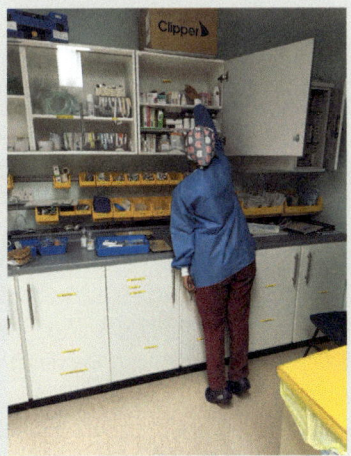

A drug cupboard – or any cupboard – may have been installed with little consideration to the typical height of the fifth percentile population and may influence how easily items can be reached or seen. What if the cupboard stores medication and is above the eyeline of the individual? The reliability of selection could be influenced, especially if the area is not well lit (see later in this chapter). Over-reaching and lifting heavier objects above shoulder height are both scenarios that may cause shoulder and back injuries. Hence, if the cupboard content has not been considered, this may become a problem for staff and patient safety.

Patient falls are a well-recognised risk for most healthcare or community social care settings. Considering how the environment supports the tasks and activities that are likely to be required by patients may reveal how the environment either supports or hinders different patient or service-user groups. Examples include the reach distance of handles, direction for the opening of doors, accessibility of furniture or equipment, adequate space or a layout to accommodate typical activities, which may rely on equipment.

Addressing the risk of falls in any care setting is one of the ongoing challenges in healthcare. Observing typical patterns of movement within and interactions between people using a healthcare environment can reveal the way people 'work' or typically function there. Small adjustments in positions or layouts of an environment can be very effective to improve the safety and use of environments. For example, the bilateral positioning of toilet rolls in a stroke unit, the use of tactile cues in environments where patients may be typically visually challenged, strategically placed grab rails at frequent fall sites. This may seem like common sense but often many assumptions are made about how people will use an environment, without doing observational work to understand how different people with different needs actually use the environment. These all provide examples of the need to consider the gap between 'work-as-imagined' and 'work-as-done'.

Considering body sizes, body position and likely physical challenges specific to the users in a given context, can assist in creating personas of typical users. These can be used to understand relevant challenges. Gender, age, disability, adult and paediatric users are just some characteristics to be considered. Anthropometric data can be used to inform how to ensure an environment can accommodate those intending to use it. These resources can be found online and can provide measurements to support the design of layouts and environments, with a need to consider the correct resource for the intended population. Consideration of the critical dimensions influential to specific tasks can influence environmental and product design to support the safety and efficiency of tasks. Critical dimensions refer to the measurement that reflects the body part with greatest influence on the performance of the task. These may include a person's field of vision and eyeline height, their reach distances, and their sitting and standing heights appropriate to support seated or upright work.

The example given in Box 6.2 highlights a problem that occurred in a Trust. This Trust was the first to employ an Ergonomist and to apply human factors through user-centred task analysis to identify physical interactions likely to impact musculoskeletal injury. This approach contributed to a 36% reduction in injury rates, and in 1999 this was conservatively estimated to equate to cost savings of €5,542,065 (approximately £4.5 million) (Hignett, 2001).

Figure 6.2 illustrates the critical anthropometric dimensions 'a' to 'd' that would need to be considered to make recommendations for the design of this type of workspace. The range between which the equipment would need to vary may depend on the difference between these dimensions and the male and female staff using this environment and equipment.

Chapter 6 The Environment

BOX 6.2 Example – investigating workplace ergonomics in a pathology department

A pathology department is struggling to manage their workload and meet the performance levels required to ensure the timely review of samples. A review of the department's data reveals a low level of staff retention and a high level of sickness and absences. A staff survey reveals dissatisfaction with workload, lack of breaks and reports of musculoskeletal discomfort during work. Observations were completed and photographs taken of equipment layout and postures adopted by a range of staff while completing microscope work.

The photographs were used to evaluate the postures required by staff to study samples. The review indicated the fixed positions of equipment required staff of different statures to modify their postures or adapt their workplaces with books and boxes to achieve the required position of the microscope eyepiece. Elbows were unsupported and typically staff may be perched on the edge of a stool to complete their tasks, which required a high level of vigilance and visual demand.

A postural analysis tool was used to provide a summary of quantitative scores of several staff postures. The number of days lost to musculoskeletal injuries or sickness and absence were costed up and used to form the business case for an improved design of breaks, workplace layout and adjustable equipment.

The dimensions for the appropriate design of different workbench heights and the variable height required for seating and microscope eyepieces were used, based on anthropometric data for the critical dimensions of eye height and supported elbow height. This ensured sufficient options were available for staff of different statures working at the same time. Adjustable equipment was proposed as the preferred solution, to be supported with education and advice to support staff in understanding how to adjust their workspace.

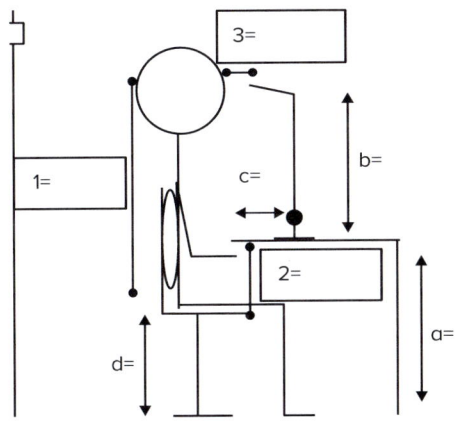

FIGURE 6.2 Critical anthropometric dimensions.

TABLE 6.1 Representative anthropometric dimensions

	Dimension description	Example adult data 5th percentile	Example adult data 95th percentile
a	Underside of elbow height to floor, sitting	male: 625.3 mm female: 584.8 mm	male: 713.6 mm female: 669.6 mm
b	Eye height to elbow	male: 544.9 mm female: 497.1 mm	male: 581.1 mm female: 523.8 mm
c	Back of elbow to wrist	male: 264.7 mm female: 233.6 mm	male: 311.9 mm female: 279.5 mm
d	Back of knee height, sitting	male: 307 mm female: 364 mm	male: 438 mm female: 478 mm

The anthropometric dimensions given in Table 6.1 (Peebles and Norris, 1998) were used to calculate the critical dimensions 1, 2 and 3 given in Figure 6.2. These dimensions informed the design requirements and adjustable range required during the procurement of chairs, tables and, where funding was available, adjustable microscopes.

The Rapid Upper Limb Assessment (RULA) and the Rapid Entire Body Assessment (REBA) tools (Hignett and McAtamney, 2000) could also be used to collect relative quantitative data on body postures and types of movement, for example, repetition or static force required by a work activity. Photographs of typical work postures are taken and can then be used to score typical postures. The tools allow you to calculate a final score that can be interpreted to reflect the level of risk and likelihood of musculoskeletal injury, indicating the need for intervention. This information can be useful where evidence is required to justify or support a business case to secure the support or funds from an organisation to modify an environment and the equipment within the environment. An example of the REBA scoring system can be seen in Figure 6.3 and Box 6.3, based on the technical note provided by Hignett and McAtamney (2000). RULA and REBA were both designed with healthcare in mind and are well used, with examples easily found on the internet[1] and in academic reviews (Hita-Gutiérrez et al., 2020). There are also non-healthcare examples, which offer good descriptions on how to approach the problem of assessing the risk in dynamic and more unpredictable settings (Duguid and Vosper, 2019).

Layout of the Environment

Historically, the design of hospitals has not included the involvement of human factors practitioners. The ability for organisations to consider how an environment may impact patient experience and staff performance may not have been considered equal to optimising layouts to maximise services and efficiencies. Yet, the lack of

---

[1] See for example https://ergo-plus.com/wp-content/uploads/rapid-entire-body-assessment-reba-1.png?x76333

Chapter 6 The Environment

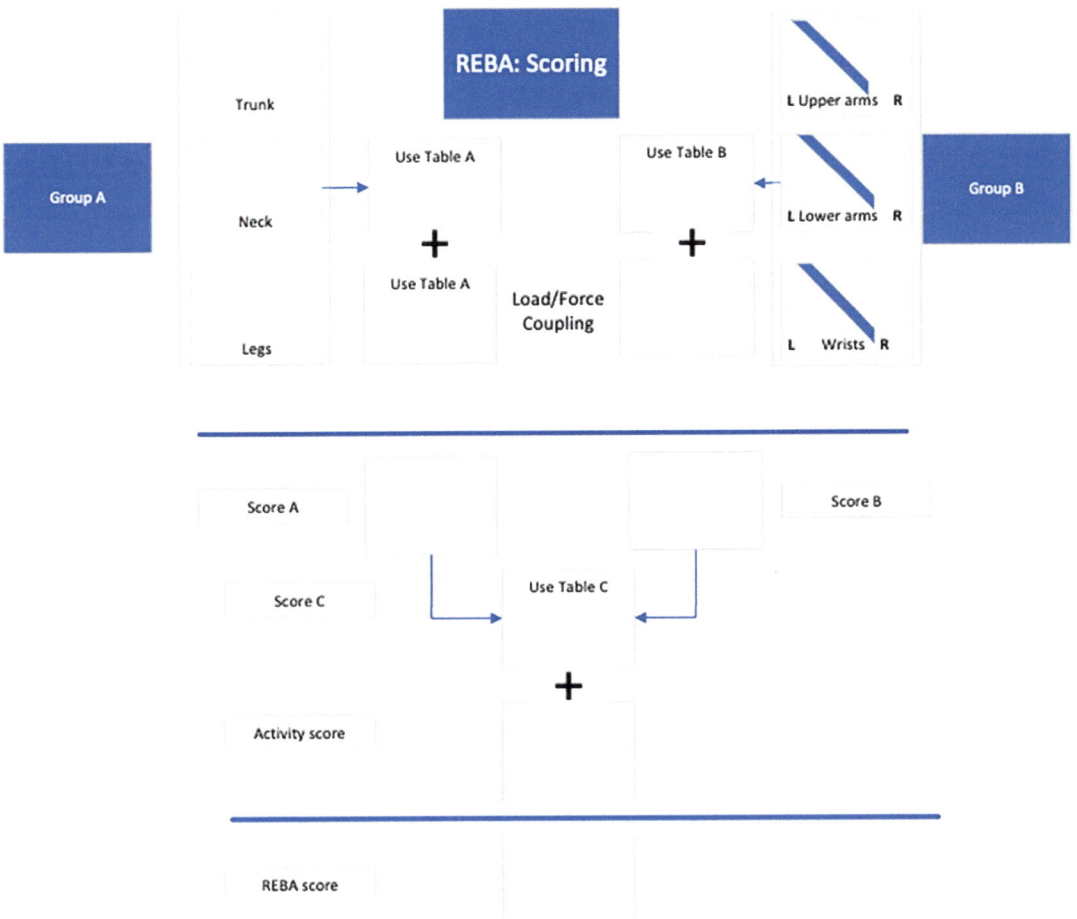

FIGURE 6.3 REBA (Rapid Entire Body Assessment) scoring system.

prioritisation of space to enable staff rest and recovery may promote fatigue and inadvertently impact staff performance, impacting the organisational effectiveness (see, for example, Chapter 4 on 'People'). Patient experience and safety can be impacted through lack of space to enable patients to process complex or difficult information or just avoid the high stress created when unable to find the department they require. Patients arriving late or anxious may impact efficiencies and safety in how engaged they can be in checks and shared decision making. It can be challenging for organisations to fully recognise how the environment may impact their core goals, and human factors could enable healthcare to seek to understand the impact.

The layout of an environment is more likely to influence how people behave or choose to complete the tasks required. Layout may include permanent fixtures and fittings, but also more adjustable items of equipment or furniture. The impact of a layout may be on the efficiency and quality of task performance, or it may have a direct impact upon the efficiency and safety of people working or experiencing the environment.

Human Factors and Ergonomics in Health and Social Care

BOX 6.3 Example – REBA (Rapid Entire Body Assessment) scoring system

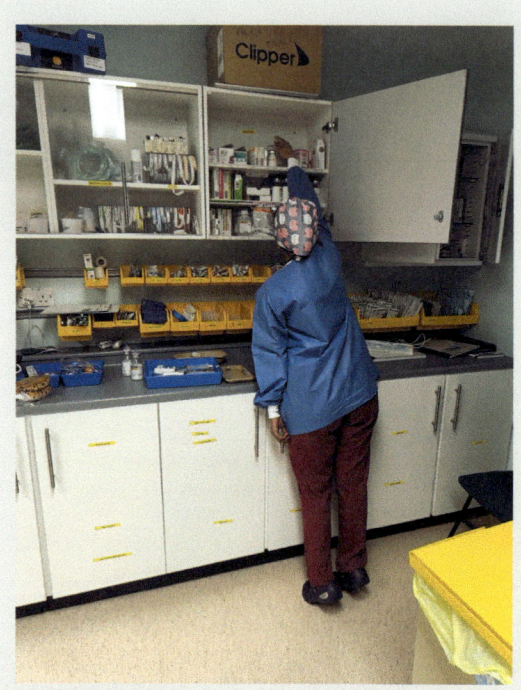

Group A
Trunk = 3
Neck = 2
Legs = 2
Total Table A = 5
Load/force coupling = 0
Score A = 5

Group B
Upper arms: L = 1 R = 5
Lower arms: L = 1 R = 2
Wrists: L = 1 R = 2
Total Table B = L = 1 R = 7
Load/force coupling = 0
Score B = 7

Score C = 8
Activity Score = 0
Score C + Activity Score = 0
REBA Score = 8

REBA risk rating
1 – negligible.
2–3 – low risk, some change may be required.
4–7 – medium risk, further investigation, change soon.
8–10 – high risk, investigate and implement change.
11+ – very high risk, implement change immediately.

A link analysis is a relatively simple method to understand and visualise the interaction between elements within the system. This may include movement or interactions of people with people, people in their environment with equipment or with the interface of a device (Stanton et al., 2013). Link analysis is used to explore the relationships between people, objects and environments, the earliest use being seen in criminal investigations. This method is strengthened when starting with a task analysis relevant to the context – this may be a work environment, computer interface or organisational department. Obtaining an accurate representation of a healthcare environment can be achieved by speaking nicely to the estates teams, who will hold blue prints of healthcare environments. There are some good examples of use of this relatively simple but effective method in healthcare settings (Davis et al., 2016). Observations of different tasks and members of staff (different colour pens can help to differentiate between roles or tasks being completed) can be recorded from lines on a map of the environment. A larger number of lines between objects required by different tasks can indicate dependency between tasks, equipment and the environment. Movement between key pieces of equipment or storage areas may indicate how work is really done and the effort or associated workload. Some interactions may highlight trade-offs that staff are more likely to adopt in time-pressured situations and these may indicate risks. Another method often used in quality improvement activities within healthcare are 'spaghetti diagrams'; these too require you to draw lines onto a representation of an environment, but typically focus on the flow and movement of people or materials often used to understand efficiencies and bottlenecks. The output of link analysis and spaghetti diagrams may look similar but each has a different focus. The link analysis seeks to understand interactions of system elements, whereas spaghetti diagrams focus on the flow of people or things in the context of an environment.

One of the greatest advantages of these methods is their simplicity and the visualisation of work in the context familiar to staff. This can provide an image to communicate between different staff groups, such as clinical staff, infection control and housekeeping staff, to enable a co-design approach to considering the options available. This basic form of tabletop modelling can also assist in the evaluation of future redesigns, before any costs are incurred, to understand how intended modifications may have unintended consequences for different users.

The simple task analysis shown in Figure 6.4 can be used to add the numbers for each task and link each number based on the likely sequence. Two different layouts are illustrated on the next page and the link analysis for layout 1 has been completed (Figure 6.5). Complete the same activity for layout 2 (Figure 6.6) and consider which layout provides the greatest efficiency, and which layout will help the reliability of the work?

You could even find your organisation's policy for taking a blood sample and consider how easy or likely it is for the policy to be adhered to in time-pressured situations. Another approach may include considering the cost associated with each link to understand the impact on staff time or physical demand and even whether this can be considered as illustrating patterns that are more or less likely to impact safety outcomes. The use of more than one method is also always an option. For example, to illustrate the physical cost calculating the REBA scores for different links may provide a cumulative and comparative view of the physical demand of one layout over another.

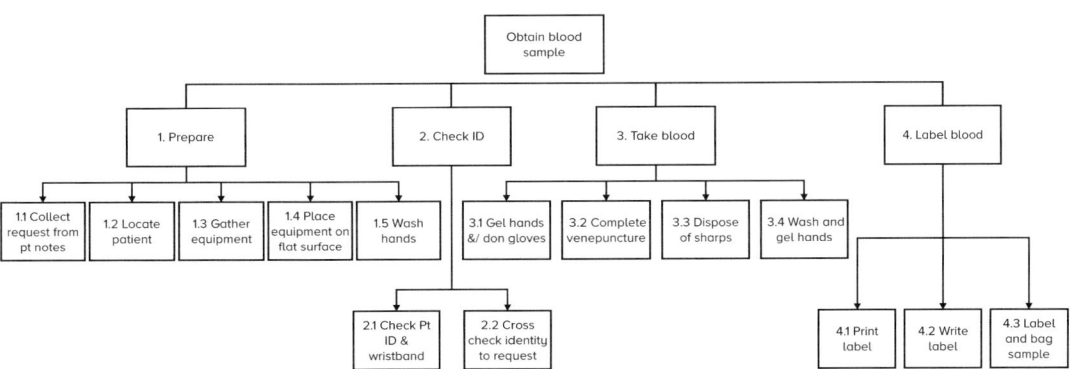

FIGURE 6.4   Hierarchical task analysis for obtaining a blood sample.

Human Factors and Ergonomics in Health and Social Care

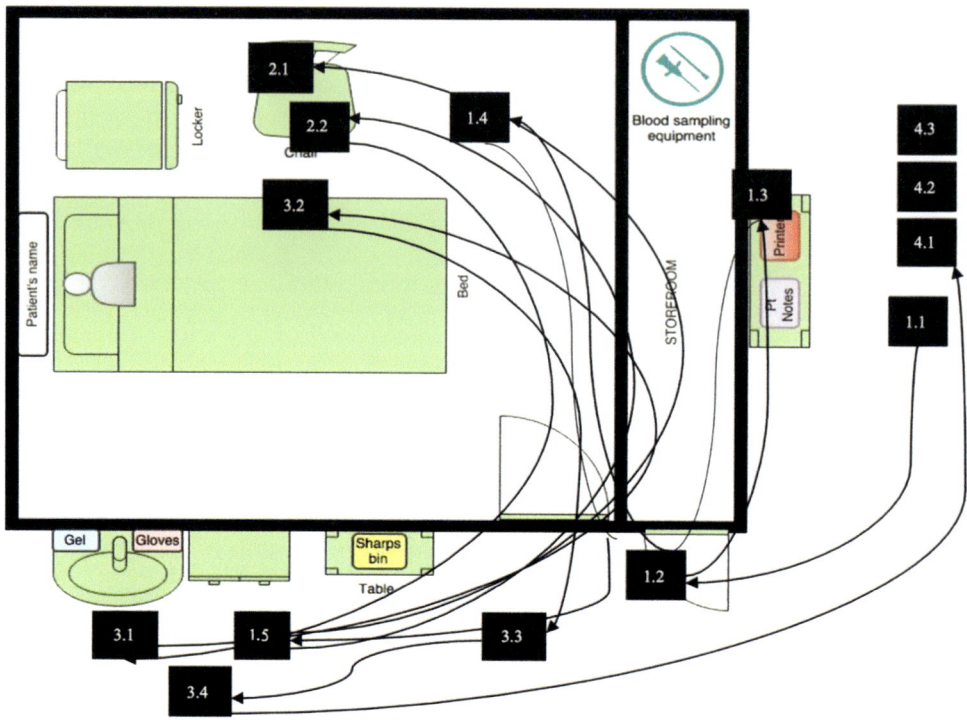

FIGURE 6.5 Link analysis example: Layout 1.

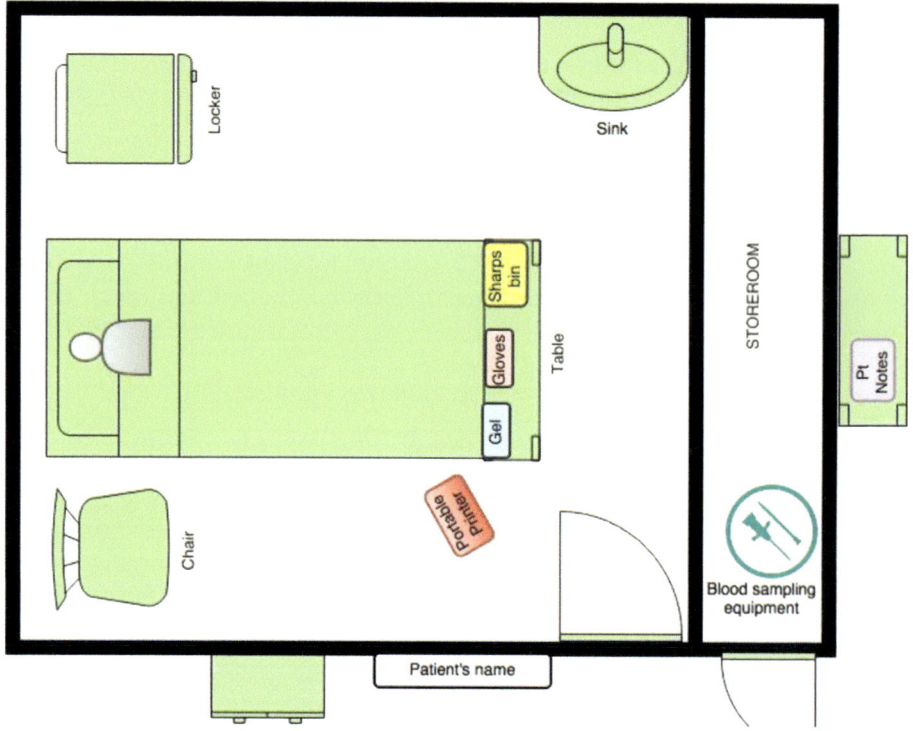

FIGURE 6.6 Layout 2 for link analysis activity.

The storage of equipment is critical to the reliability of tasks, or the order tasks are completed in. When staff are required to accurately identify and retrieve equipment, then the storage location or availability can influence patient safety, staff workload, and the stress and well-being of both patients and staff. The storage of equipment or medication in healthcare environments is often overlooked when considering how to improve safety. The responsibility for the design and approach to storage may be left to non-clinical staff, and unintended consequences may occur without an understanding of likely errors, for example look-alike labels, frequency of use or equipment commonly used together or in time-critical situations.

Human Performance Relative to the Environment

The following sections will outline how properties of the environment may influence performance and safety in an environment. The properties to be considered include noise (acoustic and auditory), lighting and temperature.

The Acoustic and Auditory Environment

Sounds can have a variety of important positive and negative effects on performance. Box 6.4 provides an example from an intensive care unit during COVID-19. Every moment – whether we are asleep or awake – auditory signals are constantly being received and processed by our auditory system to make us alert to important cues in the world, while ignoring others. Our ear drums move in response to fast and subtle variations in sound pressure, which are converted in the cochlear to electrical signals that are then sent deeper into our brains for processing.

BOX 6.4 Noise exposure in an intensive care unit during COVID-19

> Noise can be an unintended consequence of other actions, as seen in the report of an investigation completed in an adult intensive care unit during the COVID-19 pandemic (HSSIB, 2022). An industrial-sized ventilation system was in place within the unit and the investigation found that the noise at the bedside and within the unit was at a significantly high level. This was found to create challenges with communication, further exacerbated by staff being required to wear face masks. The patient was also noted to have hearing loss and immediately requested his hearing aid in the intensive care environment. This investigation suggested that noise had the potential to create distraction and impact staff attention, judgement and decision making. This example illustrates how managing one risk may introduce other environmental risks, which, if staff are unaware of the impact on human performance, can go unnoticed, with staff and patients absorbing this risk as they attempt to accommodate work environments.

Auditory Processing

Unlike being able to direct attention to visual objects with physical movements of our eyes, one of the most remarkable properties of our auditory system is in helping us direct attention to information that is important while ignoring information that is not.

The 'cocktail party' effect is a profound demonstration of how powerful our auditory system is. Imagine you are at a noisy party, having a conversation with a friend next to you. Despite all the hubbub, or maybe with a little trouble, you can understand what you are both saying, because you are able to concentrate on their voice. Suddenly your attention is drawn away from your friend to someone across the room who has just mentioned your name. This demonstrates that your auditory system, all the time, is trying to parse out uninteresting auditory signals, while monitoring important cues that are then brought to your conscious attention – much like your visual attention might be drawn to a flashing light.

Our auditory system also is very powerful for providing location cues that help us to identify sound sources. Azimuthal (left/right) localisation is achieved through a combination of timing and level differences between your two ears. Sounds on the left will arrive sooner, and louder in your left ear. Front/back and elevation judgements are less precise. Since our auditory system uses location cues to group signals and thus allow the direction of auditory attention, the ability to locate a sound is related to how intelligible it can be.

Sound Intensity and Spectrum

Noise intensity or power is usually measured in decibels (dB), which is a logarithmic scale that means that with every rise of 6 dB, sound energy is doubled. Sometimes sound spectral weightings such as dB(A) may be applied to reflect the response of the human ear more closely, which is differentially sensitive at different frequencies.

The power of sound is distributed across different frequencies, from around 40 Hz (a very low bass tone) to up to around 20 kHz (an almost inaudibly high pitch), though high frequency hearing naturally drops off with age, such that most sounds we hear are around 12 kHz or below. Speech frequencies tend to be centred between 500 and 2000 Hz, though the ability to distinguish between 'F' and 'S' sounds, for example, benefit from frequencies in the range of 8–12 kHz. This is why some sources, such as telephones, that do not reproduce the higher frequencies, can create intelligibility problems.

Sound Exposure

Typically, 40 dB might be a quiet room, 60 dB an office and 75 dB a busy restaurant. Above 85 dB might be a noisy factory, and 105 dB a night club. A jet engine can be 140 dB or more, which is the point at which physical damage may occur. Because of the logarithmic nature of sound, exposures to noise can quickly have more and more serious effects. Someone experiencing 85 dB constantly for eight hours per day would be expected to eventually experience noise-induced hearing loss over a 20-year career. At 90 dB that goes down to around four hours per day for the same effect, while only around one minute of exposure at 100 dB would have similar effects. There are now apps available that can be used to record the level of sound in decibels. This can support an initial assessment to understand the impact of the level of noise when compared to recommended levels. However, perception and reported experience of people within an environment are equally important to inform any review of a healthcare environment.

Spectral Masking

One effect of frequencies is related to masking – that is, sounds of a similar frequency can interfere with one another such that the louder one at a given frequency can cover up the quieter one. This is why, in some environments where background noises are at a different frequency from those of speech, intelligibility may not be affected, while in others it may be. This also goes for alarms or other environmental cues, which can also mask each other at specific frequencies such that one may not be heard over the other.

The Acoustic Environment

Environmental acoustics can have a significant impact on our ability to detect, locate and make sense of sounds. At a distance, high frequencies drop away first, while lower frequencies transmit further. Lower frequencies can also create resonance in other objects, creating further vibrations. Highly echoic environments reflect sounds, which mix with sounds direct from the source, and this can create both location and intelligibility problems. Many hospital environments, with long corridors and large flat reflective walls and other surfaces, tend to be quite echoic, which can affect communication and the ability to locate different alarm sounds. Echoic environments can be reduced by placing absorbent materials, such as acoustic foam, on walls and ceilings at strategic points. The noise of alarms and other environmental noises can also have profound effects on the sleep patterns of patients and can be detrimental for staff attention, as it creates a distracting environment to complete and focus upon safety-critical tasks.

Lighting of Environments

Considering the lighting of an environment may not often be considered a priority at the design stage of a healthcare environment or in safety reviews. The difference in lighting will influence the performance of some tasks, which rely upon visual accuracy. The eye receives light waves, filtered by the size of the pupil, and we perceive the information obtained via the eye in the brain. Light waves are transmitted to the back of the eye in the foveal area, which is made up of cells called 'cones' that provide the accuracy to our vision but require bright lighting. In dim lighting we rely on cells called 'rods', which can differentiate different shades but provide less detail.

Lighting Requirements

The lighting of environments is well recognised as influencing physical well-being and the performance of those who work within them. Much of the work that supports this knowledge is based in industrial or commercial settings, which focus on the impact of lighting on the ability to complete tasks that are dependent upon visual accuracy. The impact of lighting and working with computers is also an area where guidance and research has informed recommendations of lighting levels.

The Health and Safety Executive (HSE n.d.a; HSE, 1997) provide a helpful overview of the key facts relevant to ensuring that the lighting fits the task and people within the environment being considered. The basic rule is the greater the detail required by a task – for example, manipulating small items, intricate activities or reading small print – the greater the lighting that will be required. Lighting is measured in Lux, so a corridor may only require 50 Lux to be comfortable and practical, while a room where writing, reading or completing manipulation of items takes place, may require a greater level of lighting, such as 350 Lux; carrying out a task that requires high levels of dexterity or viewing of text or images may require a much higher level of Lux, such as 750 Lux.

How can you find out what the level of lighting is in a particular workspace? For a very general understanding of lighting levels the use of readily available apps can provide the ability to record lighting in an environment. This is a practical approach to completing an assessment or review of an environment and understanding if lighting is a factor contributing to workplace challenges. If discomfort or staff illness is a problem, then a more specialist service may be required.

As an example of why we might want to consider lighting, we may be reviewing cases of selection errors, perhaps well-known look-alike, sound-alike medications or perhaps just the incorrect selection of equipment or labelled products; could the lighting in the storage areas be contributing to the incorrect selections? An assessment of an environment needs to consider the typical users and, with an ageing work population, where deterioration in vision is a known impact of ageing, lighting may become a greater influence on the reliability of tasks that have a high visual demand.

The Impact of Lighting on Performance and Well-being

Currently lighting is not often mentioned or perhaps not even considered in the context of healthcare performance and patient safety. Other industries have considered lighting relative to the performance of their staff, and evidence does suggest an impact on productivity and staff well-being, for instance reducing work-related headaches and compensating for the impact of circadian rhythms, especially when working at night, or even minimising the impact of the post-lunch dip (Juslén and Tenner, 2005). The challenge in healthcare is that environments do not only have the goal of ensuring the productive and safe work of staff, but also the comfort of patients. The night shift in a hospital setting is a good example of when turning down lighting is ideal to enable patients to rest; however, this confounds the clinician delivering medication or assessing patients. The use of direct and more flexible lighting sources can help to address the mismatch between different users in the same physical space. So, how many drug trolleys have their own integral lights to support drug rounds at night and to minimise patient discomfort? Guidance is available on the level of lighting required by different health settings associated with different types of tasks (Health and Safety Executive, 1997; Michigan Department of Licensing & Regulatory Affairs, 2012; Save Money Cut Carbon, n.d.) (Table 6.2).

TABLE 6.2 Examples of recommended lighting levels

Examples of clinical areas	Recommended levels of light in Lux
General lighting	100
Nursing care	300
Examination or bedside treatment	1000
Intensive care bed area	400
Operating table	10,000–160,000
Corridors	200
Stairs	150

Staff are excellent at adapting, and asking how they achieve tasks relative to the environment can be very revealing, such as nursing staff describing wearing headtorches to complete a drug round, or midwives and obstetricians using mobile phone torches to read monitoring equipment. These examples illustrate the conflict in goals for clinicians needing to complete safety-critical tasks but not wishing to disturb the patient; this is not a challenge seen in other safety-critical industries.

We should be considering the impact of lighting for all users and all tasks in any healthcare (and social care) environment. For example, how do paramedics, community healthcare staff and other roles, who must work despite their uncontrolled environments, manage their work where they are dependent upon the lighting within any environment in which they may find themselves? To understand the impact of lighting on staff well-being and patient safety requires an acknowledgement of when the reliability of a task may be threatened if adequate lighting is not available.

Temperature of Environments

Patients and staff share the same human qualities of reacting to the thermal conditions that surround them. Generally, our bodies automatically respond to control the temperature within our bodies as we strive to keep a constant body temperature. One obvious difference between staff and patients is the level of activity; usually staff are physically well and moving (although some jobs do require static postures for extended periods of time) in the workplace, compared to patients who may be more static and may have conditions that cause changes in how their body responds to temperature. A rise or fall in body temperature can have an influence on individual performance, levels of arousal or physical capability, which can reduce the reliability of cognitive work or contribute to musculoskeletal injuries.

Thermal Regulation

As 'homeotherms' (constant body temperature) we will react to our thermal environment to preserve a constant body temperature. A rise in temperature will cause vasodilation (blood vessels widen to increase blood flow) to allow blood to flow and transfer heat via the surface of the skin, and if this is not enough to reduce the body's temperature, sweating will start. In a cooler environment the opposite reaction occurs – vasoconstriction (blood vessels narrow to reduce blood flow). This will reduce the blood flow close to the skin to preserve heat and if this is not enough to protect the body's temperature, shivering will start to increase heat production within the body. These are both very well-recognised reactions; however, the impact that they have upon human performance may not always be considered. Personal preference is a further factor that will influence how different people experience and function in the same environment. The ability to regulate your body temperature can be affected by your level of control over the physical environment, clothing essential for tasks required or, in the case of patients, some medications given may have an impact on the ability to regulate their body temperature. An increased need for staff to wear plastic materials in the form of personal protective equipment is a good example of where thermal regulation may become challenging for staff and where the building environment may need to be adapted to accommodate such changes.

Requirements and Measuring Thermal Environments

There are national and international standards that consider hot and cold work environments and how to evaluate a thermal environment to avoid harm or performance issues. The UK Health and Safety Executive provide a useful collection of resources and signposting to key standards (HSE, n.d.b). The standards require an assessment of thermal comfort and environments in the context of the work or activity that is being completed. The measurement of the thermal environment can move beyond the basic thermometer in a room to include sophisticated equipment that enables measurements of what is referred to as the 'effective temperature' (ET). This is an index that considers the impact of humidity, air temperature and air movement to assess the potential for stress created by the environment. This level of assessment may be beyond the needs of most of us looking to understand whether healthcare environments are thermally acceptable for the work and people within them.

There are challenges to balancing all the needs, as highlighted, for example, in Box 6.5, to meet all organisational goals and provide a suitable environment. But why might we want to pay more attention to the thermal environment in the context of healthcare performance and patient safety?

First, we are experiencing considerable environmental changes and seeing considerable differences in the behaviour of external temperatures. This will impact existing internal environments, which may become increasingly challenging to be a patient in and for staff to work in at certain times of the year. High and low temperatures both have the potential to influence how we perform, because they will affect our cognitive and physical performance. This may impact the reliability of decisions and actions taken when completing patient-focused tasks. High levels of heat are suggested as having the greatest impact on cognitive performance for tasks that require sustained attention (vigilance), but may also influence tasks that require differing levels of attention to make sense of complex information.

Chapter 6 The Environment

BOX 6.5 Example – unresolved thermal environment challenges

> Staff are required to dress bare below the elbow for the purpose of infection prevention and control. A healthcare environment is required to be at a cooler temperature to support clinical requirements. An old ventilation system requires some minor repairs, which means there is a strong draft directed towards some staff when required to work statically at a task. This scenario presents some typical challenges that may present in healthcare environments.
>
> Although staff recognise the need to work bare below the elbow for infection prevention and control, and a lower room temperature is necessary for clinical requirements, they are experiencing thermal and musculoskeletal discomfort when working in this environment. Despite reporting the issues, no further assessment has been completed, nor have alternative work patterns, clothing and repairs been prioritised.

The evidence also suggests tasks that require choices to be made and complex psychomotor tasks (where thinking is required to decide and complete physical actions) are detrimentally affected by increased heat (Mathews et al., 2004). However, hand-eye co-ordination and reaction time remain unaffected by heat. Low levels of temperature may also have an impact on the attention, alertness and focus given to a task. However, in general there appears to be a considerable number of unknowns on how temperature influences cognitive performance.

Physical performance may be impaired or musculoskeletal injury caused if temperatures are too low. The physiological response of vasoconstriction reduces the blood flow to muscle tissue and, if levels of exertion are high, this can reduce the performance of muscles and can cause damage to muscle tissue. High levels of temperature are generally associated with fatigue, which may also impact physical capabilities.

Understanding the thermal environment may be more important in situations where staff report a problem or injury, and incident reports recognise it as an issue. Perceptions of thermal comfort, through use of subjective rating scales, should be considered when reviewing the adequacy of the temperature in an environment. Measurements of physiological response to temperature may also be used to consider the response to a thermal environment and may include the heart rate and body temperature of those using a particular environment. A basic assessment to consider if any further evaluation or assessment is required can be completed; again the UK Health and Safety Executive offer tools that could be used to support this (HSE, n.d.c.).

The Impact of Healthcare Environments on Decision Making

Typically, healthcare requires staff and patients to make many decisions during work or visits. These will range from complex clinical decisions to just deciding which corridor to follow to reach an appointment. These may seem extremely different examples, but both rely upon processing information available to the decision maker, and how this information is presented in the environment can create uncertainty or distractions. A very well-recognised theory from the mid-twentieth century, 'signal detection theory' (Tanner and Swets, 1954), explains how a decision maker must direct their attention to key information, referred to as the 'signal', and be able to distinguish this from the background 'noise', which is anything that may attract attention in the environment. A simple example of this is the patient being anxious and rushing to attend a hospital appointment. Hospital corridors cluttered with posters and notices, ranging from directions to safety warnings or instructions on which side of the corridor to walk on, all challenge the patient to identify signs useful to help them decide on the correct lift or door to take. The environment creates a high level of background 'noise', which may create an even greater challenge for certain patient groups who may have underlying conditions that challenge their ability to process information, such as dementia or learning disabilities.

Consider the same context for staff in their work environments, where posters are frequently relied upon to communicate both social functions and safety-critical messages relating to how to complete clinical tasks or escalate clinical situations. Posters may indicate where key pieces of equipment are stored, how to escalate the care of a deteriorating patient or which button *not* to press to avoid the malfunctioning of a system relied upon to deliver care or a service. The visual clutter created in healthcare environments, albeit created with the best intention of communicating information, can confuse and misdirect the attention of those trying to make decisions.

The impact of sounds in healthcare environments has been described above. It has been suggested that, without some consideration, the presence of sounds and noise can obscure 'signals' that are intended to be helpful in identifying critical or useful information in an environment that may make a difference to supporting the care delivered and patient safety.

There is also some evidence to show that higher environmental temperatures may influence vigilance, which could impede the ability to identify 'signals' in certain types of work or activities. This may be relevant to certain jobs, which require high levels of attention for long periods of time to identify a change in very similar-looking information, for example an anaesthetist continuously monitoring a patient's vital signs in a warm theatre.

The examples provided here may have different consequences for patient and staff, perhaps impacting the patient's experience or increasing the potential for risk of harm to patients. However, either may result in delays and the wrong decision, suggesting that the design of healthcare environments can have some impact on decision making. The cues available and attracting the greatest amount of attention will have an impact upon how easily people can make decisions and the certainty with which they will make the correct decision. In Chapter 5 (on 'Teamwork and Non-technical Skills'), the term 'situation awareness' has been considered as much a property of the environment and organisation as the information held in a person's head. Assessments of healthcare environments should consider the quality of the cues and information available in the context of the clutter or 'noise'. How easy is it to distinguish the right piece of information in the time available and to be certain that this is the correct information in the context of decisions being made? In hindsight, in an investigation of an event or incident, it may be easy to recognise what 'should' or 'could' have been considered. Environments need to be judged in the context of the perspective of the person trying to make sense of the information available to them at any moment in time. Considering how likely it is that information attracts the attention of a person, how the environment emphasises or steers people to look, process and act on the cues surrounding them should be considered. This can help us to understand why certain decisions made sense at the time they were made or how an environment may need to be adjusted proactively to avoid likely errors.

Environment and Potential to Influence Well-Being

Adopting a human-centred approach implies looking at people holistically, including their physical and psychological needs as living organisms and social beings. People have an innate need for connection with nature and with other living things. Enabling and strengthening this connection can have positive and restorative effects on our well-being, for example, by reducing stress and anxiety. Many of us might seek a walk in a nearby park or forest to relieve workplace stresses, or look forward to holidays in the countryside, the hills and mountains, or visits to beaches. Often, even images of these natural settings can trigger positive emotions.

Unfortunately, the reality of hospitals and healthcare settings usually provides a stark contrast to these calming natural settings, and this can contribute to workplace stress, absenteeism and dissatisfaction. HF/E, when applied to the design of spaces and the built environment, can contribute to health and well-being in healthcare settings by applying theories and methods for bringing environments to life. Three main categories or levers for such a human-centred approach to the design of the environment have been described (Browning & Ryan, 2020):

- Nature in the space: this might be the first thing we think about, for example, having plants in our office spaces to provide visual and olfactory connections with nature. However, there are other ways of bringing nature into the environment, such as the inclusion of water and water effects, allowing for natural light, and the use of natural materials for office furniture.
- Natural analogues: the use of shapes, textures and colours that occur in nature can recreate natural experiences. An example might be the use of fabrics and materials that reflect and recreate blue shades and ripples of water or waves.
- Nature of the space: this design approach aims to recreate through physical spaces natural experiences and emotions, such as social connectiveness, refuge, curiosity and peril. You might think of spaces that are open and designed to bring people together, or spaces that are sheltered and set apart while still being integrated, for example, the use of study or meeting pods within a larger office space.

Within healthcare settings, the use of a human-centred approach to the design of spaces and the physical environment can contribute to the well-being of all people. For example:

- Reduced anxiety and reduced perception of pain among patients
- Decreased stress and improved job satisfaction among staff
- Enhanced experience for visitors.

The COVID-19 pandemic, and the shifts in working patterns resulting from it, have demonstrated an increased need for, and the potential benefits of, considering HF/E in the design of our environment beyond just the hospital setting, to ensure that the places where we work are as human-compatible as possible.

Chapter Summary

In this chapter you have been introduced to ways in which the environment can impact the safety, efficiency and demands of tasks. You have been given some simple methods to apply, which can inform and communicate the demands created by different work settings and the interaction of the person, task and environment. This chapter has also introduced the influence of environmental factors and the impact these may have on human performance. This information can help you understand certain challenges faced in healthcare settings and the potential outcome on safety, efficiency and well-being of those required to work or receive care in these environments. This chapter could also be useful for the evaluation of any future design of healthcare environments.

CIEHF HF/E Competencies

Use of a human-centred approach to the design and development of systems
- Understands the role and application of HF/E principles in optimising system performance and well-being across all ages and capabilities.
- Demonstrates the ability to enhance health, safety, comfort, quality of life, attitudes, motivation, usability, effectiveness and efficiency.

Focus on how other system components and performance-influencing factors affect people
- Determines the match and the interaction between human characteristics, abilities, capacities and motivations, and the system(s), organisation, planned or existing environment, products used, equipment, work systems, machines and tasks.
- Demonstrates the use of HF/E theories, methods and tools for analysis of systems (including process), tasks, workload (physical and mental), including mental models, communication and anthropometry.

Human capabilities and limitations
- Demonstrates a working knowledge of anatomy, functional anatomy, anthropometry, physiology, pathophysiology and environmental sciences as they apply to HF/E practice.

- Understands the effects of the environment (including acoustic, thermal, visual, vibration) and individual sensory response (sight, hearing, touch, taste, smell) on human health and performance.

Application of relevant methods, tools and techniques
- Understands the theoretical and practice bases for data collection and analysis relating to HF/E.

Professional skills and behaviours
- Understands the role of HF/E in change strategies.

References

Browning, W. D. & Ryan, C. O. 2020. *Nature inside: A biophilic design guide*. Routledge.

Davis, M., Hignett, S., Hillier, S., et al. 2016. Safer anaesthetic rooms: Human factors/ergonomics analysis of work practices. *Journal of Perioperative Practice*, 26(12), 274–280.

Duguid, A. & Vosper, H. 2019. An ergonomic assessment of small boat lobster fishing. In: Charles, R. and Golightly, D. (eds.), *Contemporary ergonomics and human factors*. Chartered Institute for Ergonomics and Human Factors. https://publications.ergonomics.org.uk/publications/an-ergonomic-assessment-of-small-boat-lobster-fishing

Health and Safety Executive. n.d.a. *Human factors: Lighting, thermal comfort, working space, noise and vibration*. https://www.hse.gov.uk/humanfactors/topics/lighting.htm

Health and Safety Executive. n.d.b. *Temperature in the workplace*. https://www.hse.gov.uk/temperature/index.htm

Health and Safety Executive. n.d.c. *Thermal comfort checklist*. https://www.hse.gov.uk/temperature/assets/docs/thermal-comfort-checklist.pdf

Health and Safety Executive. 1997. *Lighting at work*. https://www.hse.gov.uk/pubns/priced/hsg38.pdf

Hignett, S. & McAtamney, L. 2000. Rapid entire body assessment (REBA). *Applied Ergonomics*, 31(2), 201–205.

Hignett, S. 2001. Embedding ergonomics in hospital culture: Top-down and bottom-up strategies. *Applied Ergonomics*, 32, 61–69.

Hita-Gutiérrez, M., Gómez-Galán, M., Díaz-Pérez, M., et al. 2020. An overview of REBA method applications in the world. *International Journal of Environmental Research and Public Health*, 17(8), 2635.

HSSIB. 2022. *The use of an appropriate flush fluid with arterial lines*. https://www.hssib.org.uk/patient-safety-investigations/the-use-of-an-appropriate-flush-fluid-with-arterial-lines/investigation-report/

Juslén, H. T. & Tenner, A. D. 2005. Mechanisms involved in enhancing human performance by changing the lighting in the industrial workplace. *International Journal of Industrial Ergonomics*, 35, 843–855.

Mathews, G., Davies, D. R., Westerman, S. J. et al. 2004. *Human performance: Cognition, stress and individual differences*. Psychology Press.

Michigan Department of Licensing & Regulatory Affairs. 2012. *Illumination for health care facilities*. https://www.michigan.gov/-/media/Project/Websites/lara/healthsystemslicensing/Folder8/2010_Illumination_Levels.pdf?rev=0d2cdfe2d1ea4fe88dbabc3cf9b588ce

NHS Digital. 2022. *NHS sickness absence rates, January 2022, provisional statistics*. https://digital.nhs.uk/data-and-information/publications/statistical/nhs-sickness-absence-rates/january-2022

Peebles, L., & Norris, B. 1998. *Adultdata: The handbook of adult anthropometric and strength measurements*: Data for design safety. Department of Trade and Industry.

Save Money Cut Carbon. n.d. *A simple guide to hospital lighting levels*. https://www.savemoneycutcarbon.com/learn-save/a-simple-guide-to-hospital-lighting-l

Stanton, N., Salmon, P. M., Rafferty, L. A., et al. 2013. *Human factors methods: A practical guide for engineering and design*. Ashgate.

Tanner, W. P., & Swets, J. A. 1954. A decision-making theory of visual detection. *Psychology Review*, 61, 401–409.

CHAPTER 7

Tools and Technologies

Chapter Objectives and Learning Outcomes

- To acknowledge and recognise how the design of the tools used by staff, patients and service users impact people, the work they do, and ultimately the organisational goals.
- To understand the importance of context: the equipment used in health and social care should be considered when reviewing the way work is done and the impact this has on outcomes (both desirable and undesirable).
- To understand how an organisation can incorporate design thinking into the implementation and evaluation of tools and technology.
- To understand the basic concepts of usability and accessibility in relation to tools and technologies.
- To be able to use simple heuristic frameworks to assess the usability of tools and technologies in the workplace.

Introduction: Understanding How the Tools We Use Influence How We Work and Deliver Care

Tools and technologies provide a means to enhance human physical and mental abilities and have been fundamental for human development. Tools can be as simple as a pencil or a checklist, or as complex as a surgical robot. The purpose of each tool or technology is to afford some advantage to the people using them. However, if people cannot use the tools, or if tools have not been designed with an understanding of how, where and when they will be used, they may not work, they may fail at unexpected times, or they may mislead their users. A technology or tool will not be as effective if it is not easy to use, or if it lulls users into a false sense of security, or if it makes work less satisfying or rewarding. The more complex and sophisticated the tools become and the more we rely upon them, especially in high-hazard environments, the more important it is that their design takes into account the diversity of users, uses and use environment.

Tools and technology are part of every area of health and social care, including paper-based patient and service-user records, IT systems, client-operated devices, interventional devices and so on. Good design features may minimise usage problems, translating into better outcomes, while design flaws that impact on usability will lead to problems in usage that, in turn, may contribute to adverse outcomes (Koppel et al., 2005). Despite the fact that we are beginning to see some HF/E involvement with health technology, we need to understand how health and social care users interact with technologies, and how organisations select, maintain and train people in those technologies; we must then extend this to consider the ways in which technology designers and developers work.

Bad designs are associated with a higher training burden, creating a barrier to their use in situations where training is limited. If a tool or technology requires significant training for successful use, then it suggests that its design is suboptimal and worthy of further investigation. Poor design also affects efficiency, workload and interaction with patients and service users. Poor designs can lead to accidents and harm, either to staff, patients or service users. Device-related harms can be varied, and they can be overlooked and instead reported as 'user error' or 'decision-making failure'. It is always worth examining devices or technologies that are implicated in accidents and adverse events because there are many safety, quality and efficiency issues that might be solved with better designs.

This chapter might be of particular use for:

- Making procurement decisions
- Commissioning IT systems, hardware and software
- Investigating incidents
- Designing and evaluating services that rely heavily on health IT.

Basic Technology Considerations

When thinking about the design of tools and technologies, it is best to consider this not as designing a product per se, but rather as designing interactions to support the way people achieve goals in their everyday working lives (Preece et al., 2015). From the perspective of interaction design, usability is not an attribute of the tool or the technology, but rather something that arises from interactions within a given context. Consider the ISO definition of usability (International Organization for Standardization, 2018):

> *Extent to which a system, product or service can be used by specified users to achieve specified goals with effectiveness, efficiency and satisfaction in a specified context of use.*

This definition highlights that usability depends on who is using a product (or tool/ technology), for what purpose and under which circumstances. Usability is, therefore, an outcome of these interactions, not an attribute of the product.

HF/E considerations related to technologies can be considered in terms of users, controls, displays, functionality, automation and affordances. Defining the users of certain technologies allows us to identify the people who need to be supported by the design.

Chapter 7 Tools and Technologies

Controls allow us to interface with technology, and displays allow us to know how those technologies are behaving. The functionality of a technology defines what it can do and how it will be used, which has important implications for people. 'Affordances' is a specialist term and refers to specific characteristics of a technology, which help us to understand how the design of the technology suggests how it will be used.

Users

The design and procurement of technologies and their integration into wider systems of work should be based on the needs of the users. Also known as stakeholders, there can be a surprising diversity in how many people come into contact with a particular technology. Not only might this be a primary user, such as a doctor or a nurse, but it might also be a range of other health and social care professionals, maintenance staff, cleaning staff, patients, service users and their families. Considering the diversity of users in the design of technology helps to ensure accessibility, usability and effectiveness. Considerations can also encompass professional expertise, physical abilities, cultural backgrounds and age groups. By adopting a user-centred design approach that actively involves a representative sample of potential users during the development process, designers can identify and address specific needs and preferences, leading to more intuitive and adaptable technologies (Norman and Draper, 1986). For instance, a device that is easy to navigate for a seasoned surgeon might present challenges for a novice nurse, just as a patient with limited dexterity or vision may struggle with interfaces designed without consideration for their constraints. Inclusive design practices contribute to equitable healthcare delivery by ensuring that all users, regardless of their unique characteristics and circumstances, can effectively utilise and benefit from the technology.

Controls

Controls are the method by which a user enables changes to a device or technology that allows them to manipulate it towards their end goal. These can come in a surprising range of forms, in terms of switches, dials, wheels, pedals, track wheels, touch screens, mice, pointers, keyboards or speech. Each has strengths and weaknesses, so when thinking about the design, procurement and use of any device, it helps to think about the tasks for which it will be used, and the environment in which it will be used. For example, a speech input may be helpful where the user might not be able to use a keyboard, but it can be easily disrupted in a noisy environment, and the commands may disrupt others. Touch screens are often easy to use, also allowing multiple gestures (such as 'pinch' to zoom in), but infection control requirements may limit the utility of touch screens. The use of gloves may also interfere with touch screens, may limit touch cues or make mis-keying more likely. A computer mouse requires a flat space to use, so in space-limited circumstances a track ball may be more appropriate. The physical layout and direction in which switches, dials and wheels are moved, and their location in relation to the things they are controlling, can also have a big impact on usability. Number pads can use a 'calculator' configuration, where the top row is 7-8-9, or a 'phone' configuration, where the top row is 1-2-3, with medical devices varying in which configuration they use, allowing for a potential mis-key. Feedback – for example, a haptic or auditory click – is also important for letting the user know when a control has been enacted. Controls must be designed for the entire range of users, taking into account the variability in skill, experience and physical abilities of the user, especially with older, cognitively or physically impaired users. Clear labelling and logical grouping of functions are design elements that contribute to a more seamless operation. In an era where technology is increasingly complex, the role of design in making these tools accessible and safe for all users is an important requirement for technology design in health and social care contexts.

Displays

Displays are the means through which the user understands what the technology is doing or showing. They provide awareness of the situation in terms of how the technology is functioning and give information about the status of tasks. As with controls, there are a surprising range of forms. Visual cues – lights or screens – are the most obvious, but auditory displays (such as alarms), tactile or haptic are also useful sensory displays modes, offering different strengths and weaknesses. Effective display design requires clear, unambiguous presentation of information that supports rapid, accurate decision making. For visual displays this includes considering the size, colour, contrast and organisation of information to ensure it is accessible to users with diverse visual acuities and under various lighting conditions and at various distances. For auditory displays, this includes the volume, spectro-temporal characteristics, such as pitch, frequency content and repetition rate, as well as the potential masking and other acoustic effects. Whereas visual displays are useful only when in the user's visual field, auditory displays can be used whichever direction the user is looking. This makes sounds especially useful for attention-grabbing warnings (such as alarms) or for the monitoring of specific parameters (pulse and blood oxygenation). However, as our senses are constantly receiving more information than we are aware of, users quickly learn to ignore information that is perceived to be irrelevant or unreliable. Thus, over time, experts learn to understand what normally is and is not important and may only perceive that information.

Functionality

Technology is used to enhance work or enable it to happen. This might be a lifting device to amplify human physical abilities or an imaging device to enhance human visual perceptual abilities to see inside the body. Increasingly, technologies have some component of automation that processes information to perform tasks in the background that will aid the users in some way. Most technologies come with an array of functions, settings and capabilities that, on one hand, can enhance human abilities in myriad ways but, on the other hand, can make a single function more difficult to use or access. This is known as the 'functionality versus usability trade-off'. That is, if a device can only perform one function, it is likely to be much easier to train people to use that than a device that can perform many different functions. For example, while many modern ventilators have a huge array of options and settings, for the vast majority of patients only a very small subset of those functions are used. Interfaces – how a user interacts with the device – have a big part to play in managing this trade-off. Your smartphone has a vast array of functions – email, text, calls, GPS, internet, apps – and has been (in most instances) carefully designed. Thus, what a device can do, how it is used, and how it is designed, all have an impact on ease-of-use, the amount of training required to use it and the likely instances of mistaken use or errors.

Chapter 7 Tools and Technologies

Automation

Automation is understandably very attractive, amplifying human abilities by taking work that humans can do and then potentially doing it faster, more reliably, more efficiently and more effectively. However, there can be some significant downsides that should also be considered. These 'ironies of automation' can be counter-intuitive and can create a range of surprises that are often hidden sources of problems, errors, costs or dissatisfaction (Bainbridge, 1983). This includes:

- De-skilling – that is, when a device takes over from a human, the human skills for performing that task degrade, so when the device is no longer available, humans can no longer perform the tasks.
- More training – rather than requiring less skill, automated systems usually require more knowledge and training to use, since there is often a need to be able to manually perform the task that is automated, and to be able to understand, manage and use the automation.
- Significant changes to the work – rather than being a simple technological substitute, replacing human work, automation usually requires significant changes to the tasks, people and roles required to complete them.
- Reduced awareness – automation can hide aspects of information and tasks that previously were much easier to perceive, resulting in less overall awareness of what is going on at any one time.
- Increase in complexity – rather than simplifying a task, automation can often add complexity simply through the increased technological features of the work that create a need to understand and manage the automation in the appropriate way.
- Exacerbates cognitive workload problems – while technologies can offload some cognitive requirements, they can also lead to increases in others (for example, a need to monitor the task and the behaviour of the technology) or can lead to greater peaks and troughs in cognitive demands – going from low demands to high demands in a short space of time – that can create new opportunities for failures.
- Under- or over-trust – users can trust the automated system so much that they fail to adequately oversee or question its outputs; or they can mistrust a device so much that it becomes unused, or is used alongside the traditional work, adding to the task demands without improving the outcomes.

Affordances

The concept of affordances refers to the qualities or features of an object that suggest how it can be used, essentially guiding the user's interactions with the tool (Norman, 2013). This design minimises the need for extensive training or instructions, enabling users to leverage the tool effectively with minimal cognitive effort. The design of scissors, with distinct finger holes and blades, inherently communicates its function and the manner of its use. Affordances suggest possibilities as to how an object might be used – in this case, the holes tell us that we should put our fingers in. The size of the holes act as a constraint: there's only room for one digit in the small hole, but room for several in the larger hole. As soon as you see your hand in close proximity to the scissors, it is immediately obvious which digits go where. It works because everything is visible, and we rapidly acquire a reasonably accurate conceptual model of what needs to happen.

A simple everyday example is doors. Doors usually only move in one direction, and to get through them you either push them or pull them. If a door needs to be pulled, there will need to be a handle on the appropriate side of the door. The presence of the handle is an affordance – it tells you to pull the door (and where to pull). A flat surface on a door is also an affordance – we would probably expect to push such a door. However, we need to know *where* to push – if you push too close to the hinges, the door won't move. A flat plate in the appropriate place would convey this information to you. You have no doubt come across examples of doors that for style reasons do not include such plates, and you have probably spent some time trying to work out where to push or found doors that have handles on both the 'pull' and 'push' sides.

Similarly, in healthcare settings, the clarity of affordances in device design directly influences the ease with which healthcare professionals can perform procedures, thereby impacting patient safety and treatment outcomes. The lack of clear affordances for correct usage can lead to problems in use, particularly under high-stress conditions where precision is critical.

Heuristics

Few people can be experts in the many different nuances of designs. To help think broadly about the usability issues you may encounter, heuristics serve as guiding principles or 'rules of thumb' that simplify decision-making processes and design considerations for developers and designers. In the context of medical technology, heuristics can help address complex user needs and environmental factors by providing straightforward approaches to usability, accessibility and safety. Frequently used are Nielsen's Usability Heuristics for User Interface Design (Nielsen, 1994):

1. *Visibility of system status.* Do you know what the equipment is doing right now? Well-designed user interfaces should make the status clear and let you know when something you have done has changed that status. This feedback needs to be prompt, and it also needs to be continuous.
2. *Match between the system and the real world.* Designs should follow real-world conventions and use, for instance, terms and icons that are likely to be universally recognised, such as mapping the flap controls to flat levers and wheel controls to circular switches in cockpit design.
3. *User control and freedom.* If a device is intuitively designed, it should be obvious how to use it – the affordances and constraints should make that clear. It is important that users can explore the use of a device through interactions, knowing that if they have done something wrong they will be able to undo it easily.
4. *Consistency and standards.* Past experience will be one element that influences how a user engages with a new piece of equipment. Going against convention increases cognitive workload and therefore makes errors more likely.
5. *Error prevention.* Good design should prevent the wrong things from happening, and ideally allow recovery before it gets to the point of no return. For example, in word-processing packages there is a prompt to save before exiting, as well as the addition of 'autosave'.

6. *Recognition rather than recall.* There is a burden on a user's workload if they have to memorise how to use a piece of technology, so prompts to trigger the correct action lead to better usability.
7. *Flexibility.* Being able to use shortcuts or personalise the interface to support more advanced working means that the device does not become frustrating for more experienced users. Flexibly designed user interfaces can also support those with impairments, for example, being able to change font sizes and colours for those with visual impairments.
8. *Aesthetic and minimalist design.* Any superfluous information on a user interface competes with critical information, making it more difficult to discern. For example, with some medication packaging, brand labelling often makes it harder to perceive safety-critical information.
9. *Help users recognise, diagnose and recover from errors.* Good user interfaces will make it clear what the error is and will lead you to a solution rather than an incomprehensible error code, for example.
10. *Help and documentation.* If the design does not contain all the information you require, you need to be able to access essential information readily. 'Help' functions need to be easy to search and should provide the user with concrete steps to solve their problem.

Instructions and Training

Frequently, when there are problems interacting with technology people ask the question 'But why didn't they just read the instruction manual?' From what we have discussed so far in this book, one obvious answer is that this demands a behavioural response to the problem, which we know from the hierarchy of controls is probably least likely to be effective. Also, there are further aspects, such as organisational and task factors, to consider – often, time to ensure that users fully understand how to use equipment just is not built into the procedures that govern work practice. It is also probably assumed that implementation of any procedure comes with training. In short, whether instruction manuals are engaged with is just another outcome of our complex sociotechnical system. When they are used, the design and development of instruction manuals and procedures is also important. Just as with the device itself, writing effective procedures and instruction manuals benefits from a user-centred systems approach. We often see procedures criticised in response to incident investigations, and rewriting is often offered as a solution to a problem.

In Chapter 3, task analysis was introduced as an HF/E approach to understand and represent the work that people do. Methods such as hierarchical task analysis (HTA) are excellent tools to help write better procedures. The output of the HTA can be converted directly into a step-by-step procedure. Furthermore, the systematic failure analysis (for example, SHERPA: Systematic Human Error Reduction and Prediction Approach) can identify particularly critical steps. These can be highlighted in the procedure (for example, with a warning symbol) and a rationale for certain steps can be provided, when the thinking might not be immediately obvious. For example, consider procedures in a nuclear power plant or a petrochemical facility, where the physical and chemical processes might require specialist knowledge not readily available to those operating the equipment. The Chartered Institute of Ergonomics and Human Factors has also published guidance on writing better procedures (CIEHF, 2020a).

Regulatory Approaches

For medical devices, as specific examples of tools and technologies, extensive regulatory guidance is available to enhance usability and safety. ISO/IEC 62366-1 (Part 1) is the international standard that describes the application of usability engineering to medical devices (International Organization for Standardization, 2015). This has been around since 2007, and it was adopted in the UK by the Medicines and Healthcare products Regulatory Agency in 2017 (updated 2021). The aim is to reduce errors relating to poor design, especially when devices have complex user interfaces. Table 7.1 shows the steps that need to be taken by medical device manufacturers in order to develop a product that is safe and effective in use.

In the United States in 2016 the Food and Drug Administration (FDA) developed guidelines to assist device designers in applying appropriate human factors and usability considerations so as to ensure devices would be safe and easy to use. This consists of identifying the users, use environments and interfaces; conducting a task analysis and then a fault analysis; using formative user trials to test these potential issues and a final summative analysis to validate the final design for approval. Thus, it consists of the basic principles of good design and usually empirical demonstration of those designs with a variety of users under realistic conditions.

TABLE 7.1 Steps recommended in usability engineering for medical devices

Stage	Elements	Notes
Creation of use specification	Who are the users? What might they use the device for? How does this relate to intended/claimed uses of the device? What environments might they be working in? How often would they use it? What training will they receive before using the device?	Observations, interviews, focus groups and questionnaires can all provide data relating to uses/users and environments. Remember that 'users' are not just frontline staff. What about, for example, engineers or cleaners? When users are identified, personas of 'typical' users (and their typical environmental contexts) can be developed.
Identification of known use problems	What data is available regarding use problems, either about this specific device or similar ones?	Sources may include internally and externally held data; also from post-market surveillance, complaints or incident reports.
Risk assessment of use and use error	What are the high-level tasks and user-interface factors that might be relevant to safety? What potential errors can you see associated with particular tasks?	Task analysis and related tools are the most useful here. HTA, walk-through talk-through, verbal protocol analysis, for example, supplemented with interviews and focus groups. Heuristic analysis is also useful.

Stage	Elements	Notes
	With which part of the task, or with which user interface characteristic, is each potential error associated? What is the potential severity of harm associated with these errors? What are the priorities (in terms of design) for risk mitigation?	The findings from your analysis (the identification of reasonably foreseeable use errors) need to be documented. Deciding which tasks/task elements are safety critical is based on risk assessment (for example, identifying hazards and associated harms or likelihood of harm being realised). The output of this allows you to identify parts of the design that need to be improved. Prioritising allows you to decide where to focus the next stage of the redesign.
Formative and summative evaluation	Formative evaluation should be ongoing throughout the design process. Device prototypes need to be assessed for meeting user need and mitigation of the potential errors identified. Formative evaluation also allows the identification of previously unidentified risks. This tweaking and testing should be an iterative process. Summative evaluation happens near the end of the design process and attempts to demonstrate that the users can operate the device in realistic contexts without error or harm. What tasks would need to be included in any evaluation to ensure that safety-critical characteristics and factors are assessed? Related to this, what are the design characteristics that attempt to mitigate any risks associated with use? Following testing, were there any user errors? Were any of these safety critical? Were any of these new errors? Is the risk posed by these errors acceptable? Does the design need to be modified?	Ideally, you should test all hazard-related tasks, or at least the ones that are deemed to have the highest risk of harm. Evaluation needs to be planned and documented. Planning takes the form of a user interface specification. This should capture the design characteristics that are intended to prevent use error (such as button shape, colour, use of alarms, for example). The evaluation plan should then relate to this specification: which design characteristics are being tested during each evaluation? Think back to your use specification: who will be using the device, and in what environments? Testing needs to reflect these users and contexts. You need to justify the rationale for your testing plan: this includes the number of testers. You will also need ethical approval for testing. Document findings of testing, risk assessing any new use errors identified. Design modification and formative testing should continue until you are satisfied that the device is safe in use. At this stage, the design is fixed and can now be tested summatively.

(continued)

TABLE 7.1 (*Continued*)

Stage	Elements	Notes
Training	What knowledge and skills do your users need to safely interact with the device? Are they likely to have this? What training will be necessary?	How will training be delivered? You need to think about whether this is reasonable for all the contexts of use you have considered. For example, care often involves bank staff – will they have access to the required training? Test the training: does the training deliver what you expected in terms of supporting performance.
Final reporting	This takes the form of a human factors summary report.	It includes: • Users/uses/environments • Required training • Summary of known use problems • Risk assessment (and how this was used to identify and prioritise task selection) • Summary of formative evaluation • Results of summative evaluation • Risk–benefit analysis • Conclusions
Post-market surveillance	How will you know how the device performs in the real world?	Manufacturers require a systematic approach to this. They must actively seek user feedback on their devices. This needs to be a two-way process: manufacturers need to inform users when they become aware of any problems. These problems might not directly be about the specific device – if the manufacturer becomes aware of problems with similar/competitor products that might be relevant, there is a duty to disclose this as well. Adverse event data is publicly available through several resources. These must be monitored and acted upon.

Tools and Technology Design Examples

Case Study: Electronic Manual Sphygmomanometer

Consider the design of an electronic manual sphygmomanometer. It has an 'on' button, which – as we might reasonably expect as a result of transference – also acts as the 'off' button. To get the device to switch on, you need to hold the button for two seconds. However, if you hold the switch down for longer than two seconds, the device switches back off again. This may confuse some users who might expect a switch to operate immediately. Feedback on these actions is not immediately obvious. When the device is switched on, a light appears on the pressure dial. If the button is held down long enough to switch the device off, the light disappears. However, when the user first interacts with the device, they will not necessarily notice these lights – the feedback is not obviously linked to the button operation. There are other similar devices that do not have the same timing issue, but they require significant mechanical strength to operate the 'on' switch – more than might be expected from previous experience of such equipment. In both cases, a combination of negative transference, failure to understand the mapping and weak feedback often result in the user believing the equipment is not functioning.

Case Study: The Design of the Delivery System for Contraceptive Implants

Contraceptive implants are highly effective long-acting reversible contraceptives with a good safety record. Implants are inserted sub-dermally in the medial aspect of the upper arm using an applicator, such as the one shown in Figure 7.1 (Rowlands et al., 2010), which was in use until it was replaced with a redesigned device towards the end of 2010. Among the reasons for redesign were usability problems with the applicator, which could result in adverse outcomes, such as non-insertion of the implant.

Using the concepts of affordances and constraints helps reveal several problems with this design. The implant is inserted under the skin with the needle, and then the implant is deposited by holding the obturator and retracting the needle. The device

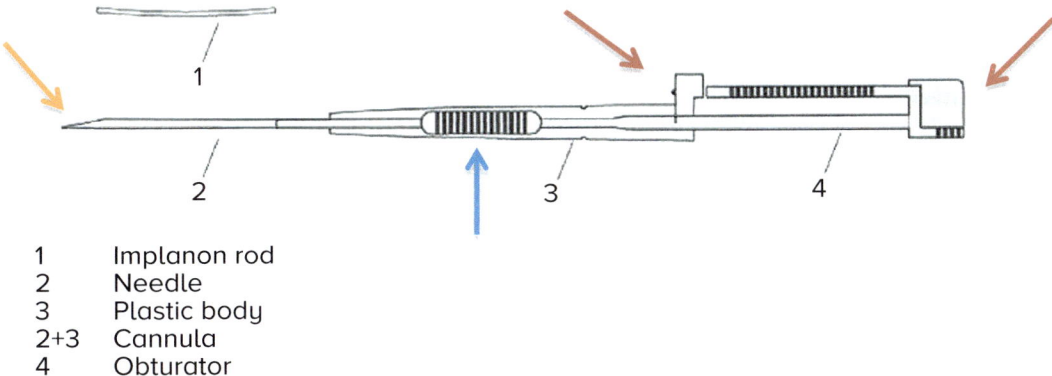

1	Implanon rod
2	Needle
3	Plastic body
2+3	Cannula
4	Obturator

FIGURE 7.1 Delivery applicator for an etonogestrel contraceptive implant.

looks rather like a syringe, and indeed this similarity may be further cemented in the mind of the healthcare practitioner by the fact the procedure would start with a subcutaneous injection of a local anaesthetic. If the applicator were to be held as if one were about to do a venepuncture, with thumb on top and fingers underneath, then it would be difficult to position the needle correctly, as it needs to lie horizontally in the sub-dermal tissue. Downwards angling of the needle might result in deep insertion. Holding the applicator incorrectly also risks pushing the obturator, rather than keeping it static, and this could result in the implant being pushed into tissues where either damage may occur, or drug delivery may be impacted.

Looking at Figure 7.1, you can see that the device has an affordance that indicates how it should be held, in the shape of the ridged grip areas either side of the cannula (indicated by the middle arrow). However, this affordance might be less strong than the unintentionally included affordances that make the device appear like a syringe (indicated by the two arrows on the right). There are also no constraints that prevent the user from holding the device in this way. In addition, holding the device like a syringe with the tip angled down *before* insertion can also lead to the implant dropping out of the needle. This would also lead to non-insertion. The implant was colourless, making it harder to notice the absence of the implant from the needle.

Later versions of the device were able to address many of these issues through better design. Radio-opacity allows the implant to be located more easily after insertion. A redesign of the applicator, with a slider on top and an indent, acts as an affordance to encourage the correct placement of the finger, which also allows single-handed operation. When held in this way, it is very difficult to angle the device in a way that would encourage deep insertion. The changes also meant that the device no longer looked like a syringe. Finally, the implant and obturator are now differently coloured, so it is also clearer when there is no implant.

Case Study: Applying HF/E Principles to the Design and Testing of Rapidly Manufactured Ventilators During the Covid-19 Pandemic

During the first wave of the pandemic, many countries shared a similar experience of a massive increase in demand for ICU facilities, and rapid need to manufacture, design and build thousands of ventilators. A summary of the guidance from the Chartered Institute of Ergonomics and Human Factors to support manufacturers through usability testing revealed the pragmatic nature of human factors that can allow rapid adaptation in a very short timeframe. This is shown in Figure 7.2 (CIEHF, 2020b).

In terms of users, additional considerations included staff working outside the scope of their normal roles, for example, staff who had no prior experience of intensive care, and the need for staff to carry out tasks while wearing significant amounts of PPE. Environmental aspects included ventilators being used outside ICU or even in completely new and untested locations. Ventilators would need to be moved, so weight was important to avoid musculoskeletal problems associated with moving and setting up. Connectors needed to work across all these different settings and be easily recognisable. Retractable cables were considered to avoid trip hazards etc. Existing procedures for three models of ventilator were used to develop task

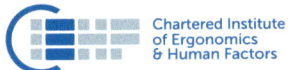

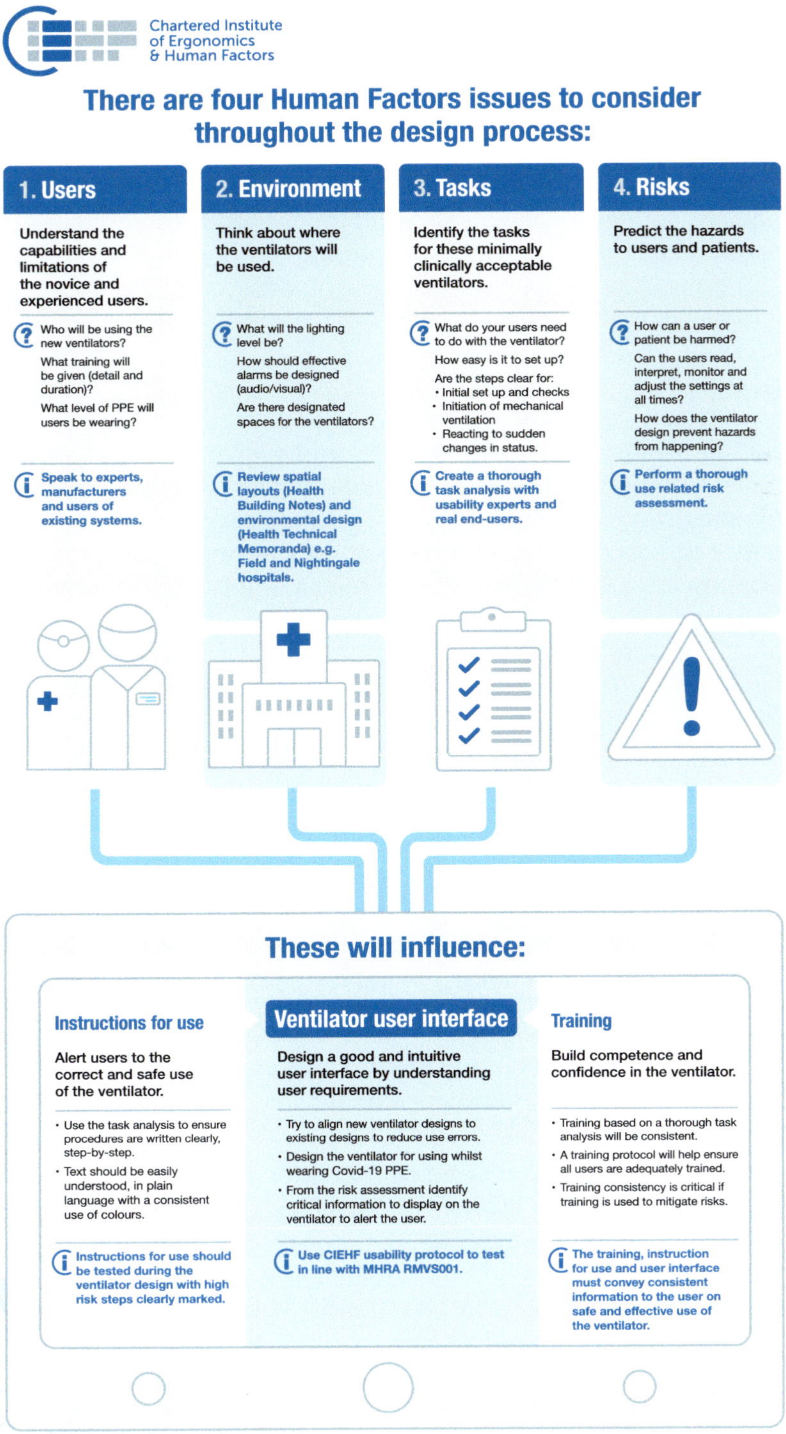

FIGURE 7.2 The CIEHF guidance for the design of rapidly manufactured ventilator systems.

Source: The Chartered Institute of Ergonomics and Human Factors. Reproduced with permission.

analyses for frequently occurring and safety-critical tasks. Errors were identified from previous research and used to both establish the task scenarios and to develop evaluation criteria. Task scenarios were supported with patient profiles to allow end-users to explore the prototype design or to carry out an online evaluation.

This approach encouraged standard designs and protocols to prevent avoidable harm to patients, while the usability testing protocol supported realistic testing (work-as-done), including operability while wearing a range of PPE. The guidance, the scenarios and the evaluation protocol were all designed as simple tools, and this approach could easily be adapted for other equipment.

Chapter Summary

Thinking about the design, work context, users and everyday use of tools and technology is important both in helping us to understand why there might be problems with an existing piece of equipment and also in determining what to look for when considering procurement of new tools and technologies. While there are many books, approaches and practices, and a vast amount of expertise in areas such as user-centred design, this chapter distilled some of the key considerations. The case studies illustrated some of the ways in which these design considerations can manifest in practice. This can help you start thinking more deeply about how you utilise tools and technologies, how they are designed, and how they fit with the environment, not just in health and social care, but all around you.

CIEHF HF/E Competencies

Use of a human-centred approach to the design and development of systems
- Understands the role and application of HF/E principles in optimising system performance and well-being across all ages and capabilities.
- Demonstrates ability to enhance health, safety, comfort, quality of life, attitudes, motivation, usability, effectiveness and efficiency.

Application of relevant methods, tools and techniques
- Understands the theoretical and practice bases for HF/E relating to design and development of systems.
- Understands the theoretical and practice bases for (re)design of human interfaces (physical and mental).
- Utilises a systems approach to the human aspects of the specification, design, assessment and acceptance of products, services and human factors interventions.

References

Bainbridge, L. 1983. Ironies of automation. *Automatica,* 19(6), 775–779. https://doi.org/http://dx.doi.org/10.1016/0005-1098(83)90046-8

CIEHF. 2020a. *Guidance on design of effective work procedures*. https://ergonomics.org.uk/resource/guidance-on-design-of-effective-work-procedures.html

CIEHF. 2020b. *Human Factors in the Design and Operation of Ventilators for Covid-19*. https://ergonomics.org.uk/resource/design-guidance-for-ventilators.html

International Organization for Standardization. 2015. ISO/IEC 62366-1:2015 Medical Devices - Part 1: Application of usability engineering to medical devices. Geneva: ISO.

International Organization for Standardization. 2018. ISO 9241-11:2018 Ergonomics of human-system interaction. Part 11: Usability: Definitions and concepts. Geneva: ISO.

Koppel, R., Metlay, J. P., Cohen, A., et al. 2005. Role of computerized physician order entry systems in facilitating medication errors. *JAMA,* 293(10), 1197–1203.

Nielsen, J. 1994. *10 Heuristics for User Interface Design*. Nielsen Norman Group. https://www.nngroup.com/articles/ten-usability-heuristics/

Norman, D. A. & Draper, S. W. 1986. *User Centered System Design; New Perspectives on Human-Computer Interaction*. L. Erlbaum Associates Inc.

Norman, D. 2013. *The Design of Everyday Things: revised and expanded edition*. MIT Press.

Preece, J., Rogers, Y. & Sharp, H. 2015. *Interaction Design: Beyond human-computer interaction*. John Wiley & Sons.

Rowlands, S., Sujan, M. A. & Cooke, M. 2010. A risk management approach to the design of contraceptive implants. *Journal of Family Planning and Reproductive Health Care,* 36(4), 191–195.

CHAPTER 8
Applying Human Factors/Ergonomics to Understanding Outcomes

Chapter Objectives and Learning Outcomes

- To describe different types of outcomes.
- To explain how outcomes are produced by interactions of elements of the work system.
- To describe principles for measurement and monitoring of outcomes.

Introduction: What Matters and How Do We Know How We Are Doing?

In health and social care our primary goal is to provide high-quality care to patients to prevent or treat health conditions and support service users. A human factors and ergonomics (HF/E) approach includes such system performance outcomes but complements these with an additional focus on human well-being, both in its own right, and because the well-being of people working in a system has an impact on how well the system can perform. Consequently, HF/E is usually described as having the 'twin aims' of improving system performance and enhancing human well-being.

These twin aims are reflected in the 'outcomes' part of SEIPS (the Systems Engineering Initiative for Patient Safety) (Holden et al., 2013). The framework encourages us to consider system or organisational outcomes, patient (or service-user) outcomes and staff outcomes. In addition, some outcomes can be immediate (proximal), and other outcomes can be further in the future (distal). What outcomes are of particular relevance will depend on the system under consideration, but it is important to look at the different categories of outcomes.

In health and social care, we mostly succeed in delivering good outcomes for patients and service users, but there are limits to what we can achieve, and often different outcomes are traded off against one another. We see this, for example, in poor staff outcomes due to excessive overtime and lack of adequate rest and recovery periods in order to meet other performance-related outcomes. Knowing how – and how well – we are doing across the breadth of outcomes is critical for understanding what we might be doing right and where we might need to improve. Being able to test new ways to do things by comparing outcomes before and after a change can help us understand what works and what doesn't.

In this chapter we will look at outcomes in terms of the different types of outcomes we might consider (that is, identifying what matters) and with respect to how we might measure and monitor outcomes to enable us to understand how well we are doing. We revisit the SEIPS model to contextualise the concept of outcomes and describe different types of outcomes, consider how outcomes are shaped by interactions of the elements of the work system, and reflect on principles for measurement and monitoring. This might help you with, for example:

- Assessment of current system performance
- Investigation of patient safety incidents
- Policy and procedure development
- Evaluating the impact of improvement interventions.

Identifying Different Types of Outcomes in a Specific Context

The SEIPS model is purposefully likened to the form of the well-known Donabedian model, developed in the 1960s, for evaluating the quality of care (Donabedian, 1988). Donabedian highlighted that a single measure of quality (of medical care) focusing on patient outcomes was unrealistic. For example, some outcomes, such as mortality, might be easily measurable but fail to identify suboptimal care not resulting in death; other outcomes, such as patient experience, might not be easily measurable; and yet other outcomes might not reflect patient preferences (for example, end of life care). Therefore, Donabedian's model suggests looking at outcomes, as well as at how well effective processes are delivered, and whether there is an appropriate organisational structure in place to support this. Within SEIPS, the vague concept of 'structure' is replaced with HF/E theory in terms of the interactions of the elements of the work system. The previous chapters have covered these in detail.

Bearing in mind the twin aims of HF/E, we can identify different types of outcomes, which should be considered, albeit not as the only category of measures or indicators, in line with Donabedian's model. SEIPS, for example, suggests consideration of patient outcomes, professional (that is, staff-related) outcomes and organisational outcomes. We can identify both desirable outcomes, such as patient experience, job satisfaction and compliance with regulations, as well as undesirable outcomes, including adverse events, burnout and poor safety culture. Further, some outcomes can be observed immediately, such as an adverse drug reaction or staff stress levels, whereas other outcomes might emerge over time, such as financial impact on patients who have suffered an adverse event or the financial performance of the organisation. Table 8.1 provides further examples (see also Holden et al., 2013).

Different outcomes will be relevant for specific settings and situations, and you need to consider which outcomes are most meaningful to be captured. Needless to say, there is a risk of measurement overload. For example, it has been suggested that the US National Quality Forum catalogue consists of more than 1,100 quality indicators (Marang-van de Mheen and Vincent, 2023). Typical HF/E projects tend to focus on a much smaller number of salient and relevant outcomes. Box 8.1 provides an example of some of the outcomes that might be relevant in the design of a community diagnostic centre.

Chapter 8 Applying Human Factors/Ergonomics to Understanding Outcomes

TABLE 8.1 Examples of patient, professional and organisational outcomes (based on Holden et al., 2013)

	Patient outcomes	Professional outcomes	Organisational outcomes
Proximal	Adverse events Patient experience Patient engagement Treatment adherence Quality of care	Knowledge and skills application Adherence to protocols and procedures Teamwork effectiveness Stress Fatigue	Staffing levels Regulatory compliance Adverse event rates Process efficiency Resource utilisation
Distal	Functional limitations Long-term health status Work productivity Social isolation Overall well-being	Staff burnout Work-related injuries and illnesses Staff engagement Professional development Job satisfaction	Staff turnover Financial performance Regulatory performance Public perception Culture

BOX 8.1 Examples of system outcomes and well-being outcomes in the design of a community diagnostic centre

> Interviews were undertaken with staff working at a community hospital, providing cardiac diagnostic services such as echocardiogram. The interviews provided insights into a range of system outcomes and well-being outcomes, which staff were particularly concerned about or which they felt were important to them. These are examples rather than an exhaustive list.
>
> **System outcomes:**
> - Patient flow
> - Did not attend rates
> - Diagnostic equipment usage rates
> - Diagnostic efficiency
>
> **Well-being outcomes:**
> - Patient experience
> - Job satisfaction
> - Fatigue
> - Career progression
> - Physical security on the job
> - Valuing staff
> - Musculoskeletal disease

Impact of Interactions on Outcomes

Throughout this book we have considered how a health and social care system, and the people in it, are constantly balancing and re-balancing resources to deliver changing goals. With SEIPS, we can investigate and visualise how the observed outcomes emerge from processes, which are delivered by dynamically changing interactions of the elements of the work system, that is, the organisational environment, the tasks, the people, the physical environment, the tools and technologies, and the external environment. Outcomes are important indicators, but these need to be linked back to processes and interactions at the level of the work system in order to design improvement interventions.

If you have been reading the book sequentially, at this point you should be able to provide examples of how interactions of elements of the work system might affect outcomes. The organisational environment, the culture within an organisation, the priorities and targets and the financial situation all affect how work is designed, managed and evaluated. A culture of blame can lead to fear of disclosing incidents or talking about necessary adaptations. Inadequate and unsafe staffing levels can lead to stress, fatigue, increased number of errors and, ultimately, burnout.

The design of tasks has a critical impact on task success and error rates, which in turn is affected by the organisational environment. We could imagine forward-looking organisations in health and social care recognising the value of HF/E and employing suitably qualified practitioners, who can advise on issues such as task clarity, task complexity, workload and suitability of procedures and work instructions.

People need to feel valued at work, and they need opportunities to practise and develop their skills. Inadequate skills, knowledge and experience of staff can contribute to errors, which is exacerbated by high staff turnover due to fatigue, burnout and job dissatisfaction. The importance of effective teamwork and communication for achieving successful outcomes and delivering safe care has been frequently highlighted. Poor communication and unclear communication protocols can hinder effective co-ordination and can lead to communication breakdowns and adverse events.

The physical environment, though often neglected, can have a significant impact on outcomes. Poor lighting, excessive noise, and lack of space can affect staff health and contribute to inefficiencies and errors. The design of the physical environment can also support or hinder effective communication and relationship building. Purposeful design of physical spaces can have a positive impact on staff well-being and patient experience.

Lack of usability of tools and technologies, and misleading user interfaces, have frequently been identified as contributory factors in adverse events. Badly designed IT can lead to frustration, inefficiency and, with increasing connectivity, significant organisation-wide errors.

Lastly, the external environment sets system-wide priorities, often controls funding streams, and develops policy and plans that have longer-term impacts. These tend to have significant impact, for example, on the availability of qualified staff, the attractiveness of health and social care as a profession, and the resources available.

Chapter 8   Applying Human Factors/Ergonomics to Understanding Outcomes

The important issue to remind ourselves of is that the influence is mutual and bi-directional, that is, interactions of the elements of the work system shape outcomes, and, in turn, outcomes produce adaptations and changes, which shape how work is carried out. An example is provided in Box 8.2.

BOX 8.2   Consideration of multi-faceted outcomes in the design of community diagnostic centres

> Measures of the systems outcomes described above for a community diagnostic centre, such as diagnostic efficiency, indicated that the system was unable to manage demand, leading to a significant diagnostic backlog. Contributory factors identified included lack of diagnostic equipment and lack of suitably qualified staff. Having secured funding, a plan was drawn up for the purchase of additional equipment and for recruitment of staff.
>
> However, the success of this was limited due to the lack of physical space to accommodate the additional equipment. In addition, staff recruitment and retention proved difficult due to limited opportunities for career progression in community settings. Further, both staff and patients experienced the physical location and the transportation links as inadequate. These issues are reflected in outcomes related to staff well-being and patient experience.
>
> Understanding the breadth of outcomes, and how these are shaped by interactions of the elements of the work system, can provide more suitable levers for systems-based redesign.

Measurement and Monitoring of Outcomes

Measurement and monitoring of outcomes in health and social care is often linked closely to targets. However, when measures turn into targets, they often lose their ability to provide meaningful insights into how a system works and performs. Instead, targets and meeting targets become an end in themselves, which can even have detrimental effects on outcomes (Edwards and Black, 2023).

In the NHS there are numerous well-documented examples of the unintended consequences of outcomes as targets. The Accident & Emergency waiting time target, which suggests that 95% of patients attending the emergency department should be admitted, transferred or discharged within four hours, has sometimes led to gaming behaviours (Trivedy, 2020). These include discharging patients quickly, with potential subsequent reattendance; admitting patients to intermediate observation units, which, in effect, function as an extension of the emergency department; or admitting patients nearing the four-hour target even if their presenting condition might not necessarily justify admission. There have also been additional pressures on staff to meet the target, increasing stress and contributing to ill health and burnout.

When thinking about what outcomes to focus on and how to measure and monitor these, a few general guiding principles are helpful (Box 8.3). For complex outcomes,

BOX 8.3 Guiding principles for the measurement and monitoring of outcomes

1. There is no single measure for complex outcomes.
2. Use a variety of data sources, both quantitative and qualitative.
3. Include meaningful insights from patients and service users, families and staff.
4. Measures require clarity and purpose.
5. Be mindful of interdependencies of measures.
6. Be aware of unintended consequences.

BOX 8.4 Quantitative versus qualitative data

Data are often defined as either quantitative or qualitative. Quantitative data are numerical, and represent a single dimension that can be counted, plotted on a graph, compared with other metrics, studied over time or statistically analysed. The nature of quantification means that qualities will be lost, and care must be taken with the underlying assumptions about the model of quantification used. Qualitative data tend to come in the form of text – interviews, statements or descriptions – and so are much richer, but cannot easily be statistically manipulated. Sometimes it is not possible to measure something easily. Quantitative data alone are generally meaningless. They only become valuable when we are able to relate the numbers to something useful that they are measuring. Qualitative data contain the meaning within them. With both forms of data, failing to ask the right questions or gathering and analysing the data without carefully considering what you are doing, can lead to low quality or misleading data.

such as quality and safety, there is no single measure. Instead, we need to consider a variety of data sources, often qualitative as well as quantitative (Box 8.4). Outcome measures should consider not only what can be measured readily but should also include meaningful insight from patients and service users, their families and staff. Any measures require clarity and purpose, that is, we need to understand what we measure and why, how these measures relate to the outcome and the underlying work system. Measures can also be interdependent, which can potentially lead to false assumptions and interpretations. And, last, we need to be mindful of perverse incentives, gaming behaviours and potentially unanticipated and unintended consequences of measures.

A common problem with measures, particularly in healthcare environments, is trusting the accuracy of numerical data instead of recognising the complexity and ambiguity inherent in their generation. Very precise measures may not be representative of the system. Thus, every measure should be considered within the limitations of collection and inference, and it is highly advisable to collect data from multiple different sources, rather than relying on one measure alone. Individual measures are not independent of the wider system – so, for example, length of stay may reduce as the number of patients waiting for admission increases, rather than

Chapter 8 Applying Human Factors/Ergonomics to Understanding Outcomes

the quality of care they receive when they are there; while a shorter length of stay may also lead to patients leaving hospital too soon, and a consequent increase in readmissions. Thus, decreased length of stay does not necessarily mean better care, while a focus on reducing readmissions alone without understanding the cause (in the increased demand for beds) would lead to the wrong solutions.

Consider as a specific example the measurement and monitoring of patient safety. In the past this has typically focused on counting the number of adverse events. In the 1980s, the now well-known Harvard Medical Practice Study demonstrated, using retrospective case note reviews, that a significant number of patients admitted to hospital suffer an adverse event (Brennan et al., 1991). While this study did not set out to 'measure' patient safety, the study design has been replicated in many health systems across the world. For example, in the NHS a frequently quoted figure is that about one in ten patients admitted to a hospital suffers an adverse event, and about half of these are thought to be preventable (Vincent et al., 2001). While such studies have been instrumental in the recognition of patient safety as an important topic of national and international policy, there are many problems with this approach when used to measure patient safety (Vincent and Amalberti, 2015). Arguably, the most important among these is that such measures of past harm do not provide any indication as to how systems work and how improvements should be designed.

Vincent et al. (2014) proposed a broader framework for the measurement and monitoring of patient safety. The frequency of harm events is an important system outcome, but the framework highlights that measurement and monitoring of patient safety should tap into a broader range of data sources, providing important insights into the complex nature of patient safety as an emergent outcome. The framework consists of five dimensions as shown in Table 8.2.

TABLE 8.2 The five dimensions of the framework for measurement and monitoring of patient safety

Dimension	Description
Past harm	Has care been safe in the past? Focus on measures of past harm, for example, incidence of adverse events.
Reliability	Are care processes delivered reliably? Focus on audits and compliance rates, for example, completeness of documentation.
Sensitivity to operations	Is care safe today? Focus on understanding how well the system manages everyday changes in demand and capacity, for example, daily briefings and huddles, and involving patients in patient safety.
Anticipation and preparedness	Is care going to be safe in the future? Focus on identifying risks and strengthening the ability to respond to changes.
Integration and learning	Is effective learning from experience taking place? Focus on understanding everyday work, how interactions of the elements of the work system shape outcomes, and changes that can be made.

Measurement Futures

The future of health and social care is likely to be closely tied to the capture and analysis of data, as more health and social care work becomes digitised. The use of management science principles, with decision making based on organisational performance markers, has been increasing. The reduction in data storage costs and increasing use of digital devices means that it is possible to collect vast amounts of data. Wearable devices can collect health-related data unobtrusively for days, weeks or years. Surgical robots can measure every move a surgeon makes and provide feedback on the efficiency and safety of the surgery. Instrumented manikins can be used to feedback performance to trainees. It is possible to track people or devices as they move around the hospital. Natural language processing can be used to assess patient notes, or incident reports. This offers both incredible benefits and a range of risks.

Natural language processing is growing in use, value and specificity and can be applied to a vast range of healthcare applications, from patient notes to interview analysis and incident identification. It allows the efficient searching of large amounts of text to identify common themes or occurrences, which previously had to be sampled by hand. It can be especially powerful for exploring the free-hand treatment notes in an electronic health record to explore appropriateness of treatment, diagnostic error, or even to identify new diagnoses or treatments. Challenges are that each application requires the algorithm to be trained, which relies on a sufficient understanding of what is being sought and how that manifests within natural language. It can also over-simplify complex themes, while interpretation of the data is only as good as the models being used and the ability of the humans to interpret it.

Artificial intelligence (AI) relates to a family of statistical processing techniques that can make associations and inferences using large sets of data. There is considerable promise for this type of technology for improving prediction, prevention, diagnosis and treatment of a range of conditions (Topol, 2019). AI is already applied to radiology to help identify fractures or tumours. It can also be used to understand potential drug interactions or to create new drugs. However, AI algorithms can be opaque and can function in highly unpredictable ways outside their normal working parameters, so there is considerably more work that needs to be conducted to ensure safety and efficacy (Sujan et al., 2022).

The value of any measurement is only as good as the underlying assumptions upon which the measurement is based. Thus, simply 'crunching numbers' is likely to lead to hit-and-miss conclusions, some of which are valid and others of which may be spurious. Considerable work needs to be devoted to understanding the mechanisms of effect of different parameters and establishing more sophisticated models of performance.

Chapter Summary

In this chapter we used the SEIPS model to think about outcomes from a human factors/ergonomics perspective. The twin aims of HF/E instruct us to consider outcomes related to both system performance, as well as human well-being. SEIPS describes the different types of outcomes in terms of patient and service-user outcomes, staff outcomes and organisational outcomes. Outcomes can be both immediate as well as longer-term.

We discussed that outcomes are shaped by the interactions of the elements of the work system, that is, interactions of the organisation, the tasks, the people, the physical environment, the tools and technologies, and the external environment. In turn, looking at outcomes can provide insights into how to design interventions in the work system to improve outcomes.

The measurement and monitoring of outcomes is different from a focus on targets. Targets don't tell us how the system works, and they can lead to unintended consequences. Measurement and monitoring of outcomes should consider a broad range of data sources and include both quantitative and qualitative data.

CIEHF HF/E Competencies

Use of a human-centred approach to the design and development of systems
- Understands the role and application of HF/E principles in optimising system performance and well-being across all ages and capabilities.

Focus on how other system components and performance-influencing factors affect people
- Demonstrates a knowledge of systems theory including sociotechnical systems and culture (for example, organisational and safety culture).

Application of relevant methods, tools and techniques
- Understands the type of quantitative and qualitative data required for HF/E appraisal and design; selects and validates the proposed collection/analysis methods and tools.

References

Brennan, T. A., Leape, L. L., Laird, N. M., et al. 1991. Incidence of adverse events and negligence in hospitalized patients. *New England Journal of Medicine*, 324, 370–376.
Donabedian, A. 1988. The quality of care: How can it be assessed? *JAMA*, 260, 1743–1748.
Edwards, N. & Black, S. 2023. Targets: Unintended and unanticipated effects. *BMJ Quality & Safety*, 32, 697–699.
Holden, R. J., Carayon, P., Gurses, A. P., et al. 2013. SEIPS 2.0: A human factors framework for studying and improving the work of healthcare professionals and patients. *Ergonomics*, 56, 1669–1686.
Marang-van de Mheen, P. & Vincent, C. A. 2023. Measuring what matters: Refining our approach to quality indicators. *BMJ Quality & Safety*, 32, 305.
Sujan, M., Pool, R. & Salmon, P. 2022. Eight human factors and ergonomics principles for healthcare artificial intelligence. *BMJ Health & Care Informatics*, 29, e100516.
Topol, E. 2019. *Deep medicine: How artificial intelligence can make healthcare human again.* Hachette.
Trivedy, M. 2020. If I were minister for health, I would…review the four-hour waiting time in the emergency department. *Journal of the Royal Society of Medicine*, 114, 218–221.

Vincent, C., Neale, G. & Woloshynowych, M. 2001. Adverse events in British hospitals: Preliminary retrospective record review. *BMJ*, 322, 517–519.

Vincent, C., Burnett, S. & Carthey, J. 2014. Safety measurement and monitoring in healthcare: A framework to guide clinical teams and healthcare organisations in maintaining safety. *BMJ Quality & Safety*, 23, 670–677.

Vincent, C. & Amalberti, R. 2015. Safety in healthcare is a moving target. *BMJ Quality & Safety*, 24, 539–540.

CHAPTER 9

Organisational Learning

Chapter Objectives and Learning Outcomes

- To describe the key principles of organisational learning.
- To reflect critically on the main instruments for organisational learning used in health and social care settings.
- To describe the mindset and the practice of systems-based approaches to organisational learning.
- To relate systems-based approaches to organisational learning to current developments in healthcare.

Introduction: Improving Systems Through Learning from Experience

Successful organisations need to learn from experience; that is, they need to have the ability to identify, reflect on and embed into practice lessons from their past performance in order to enhance future performance. This ability is referred to as organisational learning. Health and social care providers need to be learning organisations in order to manage the complexity and the changing nature of care. Sustainable improvements in patient safety typically rely on adequate processes for organisational learning. Consider the prompts in Box 9.1 to help you reflect on how organisational learning works in your organisation.

In this chapter, we look at the current practice of organisational learning with a focus on patient safety. We reflect on the strengths and limitations of common approaches for organisational learning for improving patient safety. We will talk about novel frameworks and approaches to organisational learning, which highlight the importance of considering the different goals of organisational learning, and the role of the 'learner' in this process. We also describe the application of these principles for organisational learning in the recent NHS England Patient Safety Incident Response Framework (PSIRF).

BOX 9.1 Prompts for self-reflection – organisational learning in practice

- Think about how your organisation learns from experience to improve patient safety, and what kinds of processes your organisation has for this. These processes probably include, among others, formal processes such as incident reporting systems and root cause analysis.
- Next consider what your experiences are with these approaches, and to what extent they have been useful for improving patient safety.
- Finally, think about informal opportunities for learning and improving patient safety.

Organisational Learning in Healthcare

It is often suggested that the journey towards studying and improving patient safety as we know it today developed from the publication of the Institute of Medicine report 'To err is human' in 1999 in the US (Kohn et al., 2000), and the subsequent publication of the report 'An organisation with a memory' in the UK in 2000 (Department of Health, 2000). These reports built on earlier studies, including the influential Harvard Medical Practice Study (Brennan et al., 1991), and presented data that sent shockwaves through the healthcare community, policy circles and the public alike. These figures suggested that as many as 98,000 patients might die every year in the US because of healthcare errors.

From the start, these reports emphasised organisational learning within health systems. The UK report's title ('An organisation with a memory') and the subsequent 2013 Berwick report called 'A promise to learn – a commitment to act', underscore the vision of healthcare organisations dedicated to continuous learning and improvement (National Advisory Group on the Safety of Patients in England, 2013).

The literature and the concepts around organisational learning are very broad, and there is no universally agreed definition (Easterby-Smith et al., 2000). Organisational learning is sometimes described as a continuous cycle of action and reflection, which can take place at different levels, such as individual, group, organisation or even a business sector (Carroll and Edmondson, 2002). Learning in organisations can be conceptualised both as the further development and refinement of already existing knowledge and skills, as well as the collective sense making and deep reflection to qualitatively change fundamental values, beliefs and practices (Argyris and Schön, 1996). Or, in other words, to either get better at what we already do – or to reconsider what we do and to do different things in novel ways.

Compared to other safety-critical industries, there was a significant delay before healthcare started to embrace safety (that is, patient safety) as an important discipline and practice. As a result, it seemed prudent to look across domain boundaries and to take inspiration and guidance about safety practices from industries such as commercial aviation, railways, nuclear and petrochemical industries. Common safety practices across these industries include learning from incidents (LFI) and the rigorous investigation of accidents (Box 9.2). From the outset,

Chapter 9 Organisational Learning

BOX 9.2 Aviation Safety Reporting System

Among the best-known examples of incident reporting systems is the Aviation Safety Reporting System (ASRS), established in 1975 by the Federal Aviation Administration (FAA) and the National Aeronautics and Space Administration (NASA). The ASRS is often mentioned as the best practice in incident reporting, due to its long-standing duration and because it is almost unanimously regarded as a useful system by aviation stakeholders. The ASRS allows pilots, air traffic controllers and others to voluntarily share narratives of safety incidents, including near misses, equipment malfunctions and other factors contributing to risks. Reports are strictly confidential, fostering an open environment for reporting without fear of punishment. The key principles of ASRS are:

- **Confidential reporting:** Anyone involved in aviation can submit reports, just like any healthcare professional can flag safety concerns. This encourages open communication and identification of systemic issues.
- **Expert analysis:** Trained analysts, similar to healthcare safety investigators and patient safety incident response leads, review reports for immediate hazards and categorise them for further analysis. Urgent issues trigger alerts for prompt action.
- **Deeper dive:** Analysts then delve deeper, searching for underlying causes and contributing factors. This may involve contacting reporters for clarification.
- **Sharing the insights:** Analysed reports inform safety recommendations, training programmes and policy changes.

both of these safety practices have formed essential pillars of the nascent patient safety movement (Barach and Small, 2000).

Effective learning from incidents and the investigation of accidents can lead to improvements in practice, which enhance safety and productivity. The analysis of incidents and the investigation of accidents seek to reveal contributory factors and underlying causes, which can be addressed in order to reduce the likelihood of incidents and accidents recurring. Recent conceptual frameworks for learning from incidents describe this as a process that includes not only the actual investigation of incident and accident data, but also the steps that take place before and after, such as data gathering, identifying improvements, implementation and evaluation (Drupsteen and Hasle, 2014; Jacobsson et al., 2012). It is also important to consider learning as a social and organisational process, not simply a technical activity (Lukic et al., 2012). This perspective directs attention to the social and organisational enablers for effective organisational learning; that is, it is not only about the quantity and the quality of data (for example, encouraging more reporting of incidents), but, crucially, about the social infrastructure for effective organisational learning.

Healthcare policy makers integrated such safety practices from aviation and other safety-critical industries into the implementation of organisation-wide and national incident reporting systems and promoted the widespread adoption of 'root cause analysis'

(RCA) for the investigation of patient safety incidents with significant patient harm. In the NHS, the National Reporting and Learning System (NRLS) was set up in 2003 to collect and aggregate incident reporting data at a national level. NRLS built up a repository of millions of incident reports, but there is little evidence that this has contributed to any kinds of significant and sustainable improvements in patient safety (Vincent et al., 2008).

Why Are Health and Social Care Organisations Not Learning?

Given this persistent focus on promoting organisational learning in healthcare, one might anticipate substantial progress in enhancing patient safety. However, the available evidence suggests otherwise (Wears and Sutcliffe, 2019). A growing body of literature reveals that healthcare organisations continue to grapple with the challenge of translating their experiences into meaningful and lasting improvements in patient care (Kellogg et al., 2017; Macrae, 2015; Peerally et al., 2016; Sujan, 2018). Various barriers hinder effective learning from past experiences, ranging from a culture of blame to inadequate incident reporting systems, lack of feedback to staff, and the absence of visible and sustainable changes in work practices and environments (Anderson et al., 2013; Braithwaite et al., 2010; Sujan, 2015; Sujan et al., 2016a; Tucker and Edmondson, 2003). In addition, learning from incidents and the investigation of serious incidents can be perceived as contributing to the existing blame culture, because there is a temptation to focus on what individuals did wrong. The exclusive focus on these approaches as a vehicle for organisational learning also neglects other, informal learning mechanisms, such as local communities of practice (Sujan, 2015).

The breadth of these criticisms has prompted some to argue that incident reporting systems and RCA (in their current narrow implementation) are part of the problem of the lack of progress on patient safety, rather than part of the solution (Kellogg et al., 2017). In turn, these considerations have given rise to policy changes around learning from incidents and healthcare safety investigations, such as the establishment of the Health Services Safety Investigations Body (HSSIB) (Box 9.3), the Patient Safety Incident Response Framework (PSIRF) and the Learning from Patient Safety Events service (LfPSE).

BOX 9.3 Health Services Safety Investigations Body (HSSIB)

The Health Services Safety Investigations Body (HSSIB) was set up in 2016, initially as the Healthcare Safety Investigation Branch (HSIB). HSSIB is an independent safety investigation body, which has opened up a new form of organisational learning in the NHS. HSSIB receives voluntary incident reports from organisations and selects specific ones for further investigation based on national priorities and their relevance to the NHS as a whole. In the investigation process, HSSIB investigators within a multi-disciplinary team speak to people at the organisation, but also consider similar incidents and speak to stakeholders and experts more widely with the aim of moving beyond the specifics of the incident under investigation. So far, this appears to be a very promising approach for organisational learning at a national level, but through its set-up as a national body, HSSIB will most likely have limited impact on local processes for organisational learning.

Chapter 9   Organisational Learning

A New Outlook for Organisational Learning

To overcome the limitations of learning from incidents and RCA, we need to reconceptualise organisational learning (Sujan, 2022). First, we need to move beyond the narrow fixation on isolated incidents and adverse events and adopt a broader perspective that encourages learning from the entirety of everyday work. Second, we need to encourage open dialogue and collective reflection about safety rather than the more traditional dissemination of safety information based on investigations done by an individual (or a team of investigators).

Imagine, for example, a scenario where an elderly patient deteriorated at home and came to harm after they had been seen by an ambulance crew who had decided the patient would not need to be taken to the hospital. Depending on the level of harm, this incident might be investigated using traditional RCA, and the search for contributory factors and root causes would begin. Simplifying for argument's sake, the investigators would try to understand what contributed to this adverse event, and then suggest interventions to prevent it from happening again. Maybe the clinical skills of the paramedics were not sufficient, and they require additional training. Maybe the paramedics were unsure or unaware of the applicable protocols, and so these could be updated and disseminated to all paramedics. Maybe there could be more training.

What is missing here is an appreciation of how paramedics make these kinds of difficult decisions (Ingram et al., 2019). Frequently, there are other patients in the community who also require an ambulance, and paramedics need to make a trade-off whether to take a patient to hospital or whether to attend to the next emergency. Hospital emergency departments are busy places, and taking patients needlessly contributes to overcrowding and puts patients at risk. Again, a trade-off is necessary. Are there supporting services available in the local community? If so, it might be safer to leave the patient at home than to take them to an already busy emergency department.

Organisational learning for improving patient safety should seek to understand precisely such everyday trade-offs and adaptations (Sujan et al., 2016b). The purpose of organisational learning then changes from a search of what went wrong and how it might be prevented, to what kinds of trade-offs and adaptations clinicians make and how these might be supported. Recommendations and actions from this type of learning are typically not focused on the individual, but on the design of interactions of different elements of the work system, for example, by fostering trust and relationships as facilitators and enablers of adaptation; or by promoting psychological safety as a mechanism for bridging the gap between work-as-imagined and work-as-done (Sujan et al., 2019).

A corollary to this shift in focus from incidents to everyday work is that organisational learning in healthcare needs to become more social and democratic. Ownership for organisational learning frequently is allocated to a department, for example, the risk management or clinical governance department, without much involvement of frontline staff. These departments collect, analyse and distribute safety information.

The 'learning' that is generated in this way frequently consists of the dissemination of safety information without proper consideration of professional practice (Margaryan et al., 2017). However, dissemination of safety information is not the same as learning lessons and implementing these in a meaningful way in everyday practice.

In practice, many of the actual improvements take place in less formal settings, such as lunchtime working groups or interdepartmental teams that have formed temporarily around a common improvement objective. In other areas of the literature the importance of such informal communities of practice has been recognised and documented (Wenger and Snyder, 2000). Staff also need to have sufficient psychological safety to speak up and create learning in dialogue through constructive criticism of ideas and views, quite unrelated to serious incidents.

Healthcare organisations have largely failed to embrace such efforts as part of their strategies for harnessing learning to improve patient safety. Organisational learning in healthcare is still limited by the dichotomy between formal risk management efforts aimed at bringing work-as-done in line with work-as-imagined, and informal frontline efforts directed at improving everyday clinical work. The new approach to organisational learning appreciates these latter efforts and aims to embed them within the organisational learning strategy.

A Systems-Based Framework for Organisational Learning: Achieving Sustainable Change

During the COVID-19 pandemic, the Chartered Institute of Ergonomics and Human Factors (CIEHF) developed guidance on 'Achieving sustainable change: Capturing learning from COVID-19' to help organisations learn from the positive changes made as organisations adapted to the pandemic (Sujan et al., 2020). Organisations needed, and continue to need, to learn from their response to COVID-19, but deciphering the learning from such a complex situation is not straightforward. Learning from what an organisation did well is often overlooked by incident reporting systems and healthcare safety investigations that are conditioned to identify and control risks, and that focus on what went wrong. While the CIEHF guidance was developed during the pandemic, the framework for achieving sustainable change can be applied to organisational learning more broadly.

With this guidance, CIEHF drew on insights from Resilience Engineering and Safety-II (Hollnagel, 2014; Hollnagel et al., 2006). Within Safety-II, safety is regarded not as the absence of something (that is, incidents and accidents), but rather as the presence of something – the ability to anticipate and to adjust performance in order to meet changing demands and deal with disturbances and surprises. Table 9.1 provides a comparison between the traditional way of looking at safety as the absence of negative outcomes, referred to as Safety-I (or decremental safety), and the more recent Safety-II (or incremental safety) perspective. This increasingly popular perspective appears ideally suited to capture, document and learn from the many adaptations that people make during their everyday work (the 'work-as-done').

Chapter 9 Organisational Learning

TABLE 9.1 Comparison of Safety-I and Safety-II perspectives (based on Hollnagel, 2014)

Aspect	Safety-I (decremental safety)	Safety-II (incremental safety)
Definition of safety	Absence of adverse outcomes, absence of unacceptable levels of risk	Things going right, presence of resilience abilities
Safety management principle	Risk-based, control of risk through barriers	Achieving success through adaptations and trade-offs
Learning from experience	Learning from incidents and adverse outcomes, focus on root causes and contributory factors	Learning from everyday work, focus on work-as-done and trade-offs
Performance variability	Potentially harmful, constraining performance variability through standardisation and procedures	Inevitable and useful, source of success and failure

The CIEHF guidance frames organisational learning in terms of the mindset with which we approach it, and then in terms of the actions or the process to implement it (Figure 9.1). First, before we even think about what we want to learn from, we need to have clarity about what it is that we want to get out of it, so the learning goals. And they can be varied – it can be as limited as preventing a specific adverse event from recurring; or it can be about continuous improvement or identifying and responding to novel situations. The learning goals, then, determine all subsequent steps in the process. It is also important that learning is understood as consisting of more than disseminating safety information, as described above. Learning cannot be owned by a specific department. In order to be effective, organisational learning needs to actively involve the learners, and, as such, learning is for everyone. It is also important to recognise that learning is a continuous process, and it is often possible and necessary to do it at different speeds concurrently; so, an in-depth investigation can take months to complete, and the longer-term strategic interventions with the potential to make a significant difference might even require years. In the meantime, however, there might also be quick wins, fairly simple things, that might not change the system much, but that at least demonstrate that change is taking place and that there is commitment to change. Both are necessary to keep people engaged and involved. Further, depending on the learning goals, we might wish to focus on specific incidents – but if the goal is broader, to learn for continuous improvement, then we should also try and learn from a broader range of situations, so look at everyday work and try and understand how care is usually delivered successfully, and think about how this might be strengthened. And, finally, it is important to recognise that learning can be both formal and informal.

In terms of the actions, the main suggestions in the guidance are twofold: (1) it is about looking at work-as-done, the ordinary, as well as the extraordinary, which then enables us to learn about adaptations and trade-offs; (2) it is about relating these

Human Factors and Ergonomics in Health and Social Care

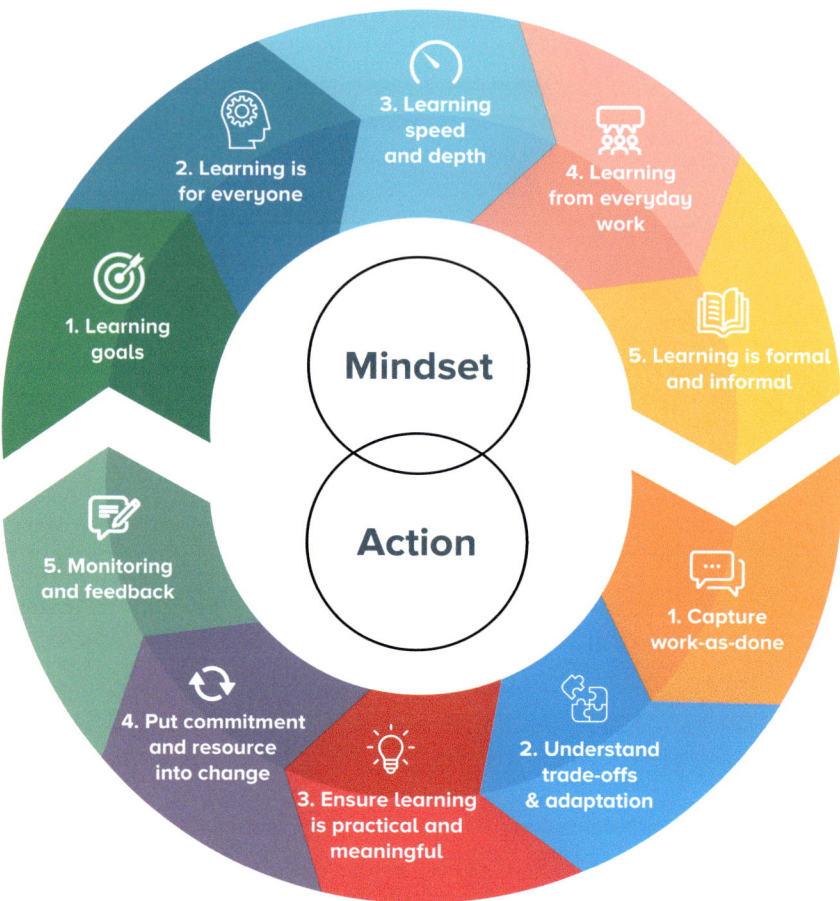

FIGURE 9.1 The CIEHF guidance on Achieving Sustainable Change
Source: Sujan et al., 2020.

insights meaningfully back to practice, which requires involvement and ownership of staff at different levels of the organisation. Organisational learning is continuous, so it is not about investigating one event thoroughly and then waiting for the next one to happen, it is a continuous process of learning from and about the system.

To get started with the practical application of the CIEHF framework for achieving sustainable change, consider the prompts in the templates given in Tables 9.2 and 9.3 (based on the templates in the guidance (Sujan et al., 2020)).

The Patient Safety Incident Response Framework

NHS England published the Patient Safety Incident Reponses Framework (PSIRF) in August 2022 to replace the existing Serious Incident Framework (SIF). The development of PSIRF was informed by critical reflection on the practical problems with healthcare safety investigations based on RCA. While, arguably, SIF has led to some improvement, it had significant limitations, including the lack of patient and family involvement, the variable and often poor quality of RCA reports, the narrow

TABLE 9.2 Mindset template with prompts

Mindset principle	Prompts
1. Learning goals	What are our learning goals?
	Do we want to learn about protocols and safeguards?
	Do we want to learn about how to make the work more flexible and responsive?
	Do we want to learn about how technology can help or hinder in becoming more efficient?
2. Learning is for everyone	Who should be involved?
	Have we identified everyone who might contribute or who might be affected?
	Are we learning at the team level, departmental level, organisational level or even wider?
	How can we involve relevant people at all levels?
3. Learning speed and depth	Have we looked at a range of options for improvement?
	Do improvements have the feel of quick fixes?
	Have we challenged ourselves and our existing beliefs?
4. Learning from everyday work	Do we focus only on adverse events and what went wrong or what could go wrong?
	Do we try to learn from everyday situations?
	Do we capture what went well and things we want to keep?
5. Learning is formal and informal	Is our learning narrowly confined to specific people or designated roles?
	How do we promote informal learning, for example, spontaneously formed working groups?
	Do we give ownership for learning and improvement to a wide range of people?
	Do we establish psychological safety for staff who contribute to change?

TABLE 9.3 Action template with prompts

Action principle	Prompts
1. Capture work-as-done	What was actually done?
	By whom?
	How is work usually done, for example, sharing of information, negotiation, delegation of tasks?
2. Understand trade-offs and adaptation	What prompted the adaptation?
	How was the need for adaptation anticipated?
	What purpose did the adaptation serve?
	What made it work/not work?

(continued)

TABLE 9.3 (continued)

Action principle	Prompts
3. Ensure learning is practical and meaningful	How do changes relate to everyday practice?
	Who should know about the changes and be involved in the design and implementation?
	Who will be affected?
	Are there any risks associated with different ways of working?
	What would help in the future?
4. Put commitment and resource into change	Who takes ownership of implementing changes?
	How do the changes improve practice, for example, does a change improve the ability to anticipate, to adapt or to make trade-offs?
	What do we need to keep an eye on related to this change?
5. Monitoring and feedback	What outcome or organisational ability do we expect to improve?
	How do we involve people to enable them to provide ongoing feedback?
	How will we make further changes?

focus on serious incidents, which disregards other potentially valuable learning opportunities, and the limited evidence of improvement in patient safety in practice. In addition, the emphasis on accountability could create a blame culture, hindering open communication and learning.

PSIRF marks a paradigm shift in how NHS organisations learn from and respond to patient safety incidents. Within PSIRF, all patient safety incidents, regardless of severity, are treated as potentially valuable sources of learning and improvement. The focus of PSIRF rebalances learning and improvement by recognising that finite resources need to be spread across learning responses, as well as practical improvements.

PSIRF builds on four foundational pillars that centre compassion and systems thinking (Box 9.4): (1) compassionate engagement and involvement of those affected by patient safety incidents; (2) application of a range of systems-based approaches to learning from patient safety incidents; (3) considered and proportionate responses to patient safety incidents; and (4) supportive oversight focusing on improvement.

In addition to the focus on learning and improvement, the first PSIRF pillar includes the concept of restorative practice (Lounsbury and Sujan, 2023). Harm from a patient safety event can be compounded inadvertently by additional harm due to the organisation's inappropriate response or lack of response and the exclusion of those impacted. For example, the independent investigation into maternity and neonatal services in two NHS hospitals in East Kent highlighted with shocking clarity how patients, family members and staff can feel invisible, insignificant, disposable,

Chapter 9 Organisational Learning

BOX 9.4 The four pillars of the Patient Safety Incident Response Framework (PSIRF)

Compassionate engagement and involvement of those affected by patient safety incidents:
Provide emotional and practical support to patients, families and staff affected by the incident. Keep them informed about the learning response process, answer questions transparently and actively listen to their concerns. Involve them in developing recommendations for improvement, empowering them to contribute to enhancing patient safety.

Application of a range of systems-based approaches to learning from patient safety incidents:
Dig deeper into the context around the actions of individuals and identify interactions among different elements of the work system that might have contributed to the incident. Consider conceptual frameworks, such as the Systems Engineering Initiative for Patient Safety (SEIPS).

Considered and proportionate responses to patient safety incidents:
Adopt a flexible approach to patient safety incident response, balancing learning and improvement. Consider the learning potential of the specific incident when selecting a learning response. Suggested tools include patient safety incident investigations, after-action reviews, multi-disciplinary team debriefings, 'swarm huddles' and thematic reviews.

Supportive oversight focusing on improvement:
Providers and oversight bodies work in collaboration. The focus is not on meeting performance and time-related targets, but improvement. Learning should take place both within an organisation, as well as across the regional and national system. The use of thematic reviews can support the sharing of learning more widely.

powerless and alienated after a patient safety incident (Kirkup, 2022). Restorative practice focuses on healing and repair of relationships following a patient safety incident (Wailling et al., 2022). The PSIRF guidance on 'Engaging and involving patients, families and staff following a patient safety incident' outlines nine principles to inform the design of organisational systems and processes for compassionate engagement. These principles include sincere apologies, individualised approaches, respect towards all impacted and clarity in the process and what to expect.

PSIRF represents a promising new framework for organisational learning in the NHS, and explicitly incorporates HF/E principles. By embracing these principles and actively engaging in organisational learning, NHS organisations, as well as others operating in the health and social care sectors, can aspire to provide safe and compassionate care to every patient and service user.

Chapter Summary

In this chapter you learnt about the criticisms of incident reporting systems and healthcare safety investigations as the predominant approaches for organisational learning. You were then introduced to a novel framework for organisational learning, based on CIEHF guidance, which describes mindset and action principles for a systems-based approach. You also encountered the practical application of systems thinking in the NHS England PSIRF. The principles described in this chapter can support you in evaluating your organisation's approach to learning and in formulating a practical roadmap for implementing a successful systems-based organisational learning approach in your own setting.

CIEHF HF/E Competencies

Focus on how other system components and performance-influencing factors affect people
- Demonstrates a knowledge of systems theory, including sociotechnical systems and culture (for example, organisational and safety culture).

Application of relevant methods, tools and techniques
- Can apply relevant legislation, codes of practice, standards (government and industry).

Demonstration of professional skills and behaviours
- Develops strategies to introduce a new design to achieve a healthy and safe human interaction.

References

Anderson, J. E., Kodate, N., Walters, R., et al. 2013. Can incident reporting improve safety? Healthcare practitioners' views of the effectiveness of incident reporting. *International Journal for Quality in Health Care*, 25, 141–150.

Argyris, C. & Schön, D. A. 1996. *Organisational learning II: Theory, method and practice*. Addison-Wesley.

Barach, P. & Small, S. D. 2000. Reporting and preventing medical mishaps: Lessons from non-medical near miss reporting systems. *BMJ*, 320, 759–763.

Braithwaite, J., Westbrook, M. T., Travaglia, J. F., et al. 2010. Cultural and associated enablers of, and barriers to, adverse incident reporting. *Quality and Safety in Health Care*, 19, 229–233.

Brennan, T. A., Leape, L. L., Laird, N. M., et al. 1991. Incidence of adverse events and negligence in hospitalized patients. *New England Journal of Medicine*, 324, 370–376.

Carroll, J. S. & Edmondson, A. C. 2002. Leading organisational learning in health care. *Quality and Safety in Health Care*, 11, 51–56.

Department of Health. 2000. *An organisation with a memory*. The Stationery Office.

Drupsteen, L. & Hasle, P. 2014. Why do organizations not learn from incidents? Bottlenecks, causes and conditions for a failure to effectively learn. *Accident Analysis and Prevention*, 72, 351–358.

Easterby-Smith, M., Crossan, M. & Nicolini, D. 2000. Organizational learning: Debates past, present and future. *Journal of Management Studies*, 37, 783–796.

Hollnagel, E. 2014. *Safety-I and Safety-II*. Ashgate.

Hollnagel, E., Woods, D. D. & Leveson, N. 2006. *Resilience engineering: Concepts and precepts*. Ashgate.

Ingram, C., Rees, N. & Sujan, M. 2019. Decision making for patients categorised as 'amber' in a rural setting. *Journal of Paramedic Practice*, 11, 239.

Jacobsson, A., Ek, Å. & Akselsson, R. 2012. Learning from incidents – A method for assessing the effectiveness of the learning cycle. *Journal of Loss Prevention in the Process Industries*, 25, 561–570.

Kellogg, K. M., Hettinger, Z., Shah, M., et al. 2017. Our current approach to root cause analysis: Is it contributing to our failure to improve patient safety? *BMJ Quality & Safety*, 26, 381–387.

Kirkup, B. 2022. *Reading the signals: Maternity and neonatal services in East Kent – the report of the independent investigation*. His Majesty's Stationery Office.

Kohn, L. T., Corrigan, J. M. & Donaldson, M. S. 2000. *To err is human: Building a safer health system*. The National Academies Press.

Lounsbury, O. & Sujan, M. 2023. Achieving a restorative Just Culture through the patient safety incident response framework. *Journal of Patient Safety and Risk Management*, 28, 153–155.

Lukic, D., Littlejohn, A. & Margaryan, A. 2012. A framework for learning from incidents in the workplace. *Safety Science*, 50, 950–957.

Macrae, C. 2015. The problem with incident reporting. *BMJ Quality & Safety*, 25, 71–75.

Margaryan, A., Littlejohn, A. & Stanton, N. A. 2017. Research and development agenda for learning from incidents. *Safety Science*, 99, 5–13.

National Advisory Group on the Safety of Patients in England. 2013. *A promise to learn – A commitment to act*. Department of Health.

Peerally, M. F., Carr, S., Waring, J., et al. 2016. The problem with root cause analysis. *BMJ Quality & Safety*, 26, 417–422.

Sujan, M. 2015. An organisation without a memory: A qualitative study of hospital staff perceptions on reporting and organisational learning for patient safety. *Reliability Engineering & System Safety*, 144, 45–52.

Sujan, M., Huang, H. & Braithwaite, J. 2016a. Why do healthcare organisations struggle to learn from experience? A Safety-II perspective. *Healthcare Systems Ergonomics and Patient Safety (HEPS)*. Conference. Toulouse.

Sujan, M., Pozzi, S. & Valbonesi, C. 2016b. Reporting and learning: From extraordinary to ordinary. In: Braithwaite, J., Wears, R. & Hollnagel, E. (eds.), *Resilient Health Care III: Reconciling work-as-imagined with work-as-done*. Ashgate.

Sujan, M. 2018. A Safety-II perspective on organisational learning in healthcare organisations: Comment on 'false dawns and new horizons in patient safety research and practice'. *International Journal of Health Policy and Management*, 7, 662–666.

Sujan, M., Huang, H. & Biggerstaff, D. 2019. Trust and psychological safety as facilitators of resilient health care. In: Braithwaite, J., Hollnagel, E. & Hunte, G. (eds.), *Resilient Health Care V: Working across boundaries*. CRC Press.

Sujan, M., Bowie, P., Smyth, M., et al. 2020. *Achieving sustainable change: Capturing lessons from COVID-19*. Chartered Institute of Ergonomics and Human Factors.

Sujan, M. 2022. Learning from everyday work: Making organisations safer by supporting staff in sharing lessons about their everyday trade-offs and adaptations. In: Nemeth, C. P. & Hollnagel, E. (eds.), *Advancing Resilient Performance*. Springer International.

Tucker, A. L. & Edmondson, A. C. 2003. Why hospitals don't learn from failures: Organizational and psychological dynamics that inhibit system change. *California Management Review*, 45, 55–72.

Vincent, C., Aylin, P., Franklin, B. D., et al. 2008. Is health care getting safer? *BMJ*, 337, a2426.

Wailling, J., Kooijman, A., Hughes, J., et al. 2022. Humanizing harm: Using a restorative approach to heal and learn from adverse events. *Health Expectations*, 25, 1192–1199.

Wears, R. & Sutcliffe, K. 2019. *Still not safe: Patient Safety and the middle-managing of American medicine*. Oxford University Press.

Wenger, E. C. & Snyder, W. M. 2000. Communities of practice: The organizational frontier. *Harvard Business Review*, 78, 139–146.

CHAPTER 10
Equality, Diversity and Inclusion

Chapter Objectives and Learning Outcomes

- To understand what is meant by the terms equality, equity, diversity and inclusion in health and social care contexts.
- To understand that protected characteristics are person factors that exist (alongside other person factors) within specific systems contexts.
- To apply systems frameworks and other HF/E tools to seek and explore diverse perspectives.
- To understand the use of participatory approaches for developing recommendations and solutions for EDI issues.
- To recognise one's own limits and perspectives.

Introduction: Designing Health and Social Care to Meet Diverse Needs

Human factors/ergonomics is in many ways a 'facilitating' science: by itself it cannot bring the change we need but applying HF/E thinking and methods can support the optimisation of all our other activity. HF/E emphasises the concept of sociotechnical systems, where the 'harder' engineered aspects interface with the 'softer' political, cultural, organisational and interpersonal elements. This is particularly important in health and social care, where much of our work is dependent on the building and maintaining of effective relationships. These relationships are not just between care professionals and patients and their families, but also between staff, and with the organisation itself.

To understand systems, we need to work with system stakeholders to consider their diverse perspectives and needs. So we need to identify our stakeholders, gather data from them and interpret it to inform our improvement strategies. However, sometimes key groups of people may be invisible to us or hiding in plain sight. Events of the past few years, such as the Black Lives Matter movement and the recognition of the extent of the influence of colonialism, are helping us realise that health and care systems, which are not designed to meet the needs of everyone, are likely to be less effective than those which do.

Focusing on equality, diversity and inclusion (EDI) is, therefore, important to achieve desired outcomes, such as safety and accessibility of services. This has recently become a key area of focus in health and social care, partly because recent events brought the extent of the problem into the spotlight. If we rewind to 2021, when the rapid development of COVID-19 vaccines gave hope that the crisis would soon be resolved, it was healthcare inequity that threatened to undermine this remarkable progress. The University of Oxford's 'Our World in Data' project revealed that (as of 23 August 2021) 32.5% of the world's population had received at least one dose of the vaccine, while 24.5% were fully vaccinated (Mathieu et al., 2020). However, these figures were driven by high-income countries that had the resources to procure vast numbers of doses in advance. On that same date, only 1.4% of low-income countries (largely those in the Global South) had received even one dose. That seemed to many people morally repugnant, especially because countries whose healthcare systems were struggling to procure vaccines were those whose healthcare systems were least likely to be able to cope with the morbidity and mortality associated with the disease.

The emergence of COVID variants highlighted the importance of vaccine equity beyond the ethical imperative. Allowing the virus to run unchecked through the Global South would act as a reservoir of new variants, some of which (as later proved) were likely to evade vaccine-induced immune responses and, therefore, threaten even fully vaccinated populations. As Dr Tedros Adhanom Ghebreyesus (Director-General of the World Health Organization) said, 'none of us will be safe until everyone is safe' (WHO, 2020).

The pandemic also highlighted diversity issues: ethnic minority groups were disproportionately affected. This was recognised and reported even very early in the pandemic. For example, in Michigan, a US state where African Americans make up only 14.1% of the population, they accounted for 33% of COVID cases and 40% of deaths (Fouad et al., 2020). Similar issues were seen around the world, and there were suggestions that genetics may contribute. However, it soon became apparent that COVID was largely amplifying something we already knew. Health status and outcomes vary widely across racial, ethnic and socioeconomic groups.

Tackling health inequalities is a wicked problem of the highest order. These issues are global as well as local, and global strategies will be required for change. It is beyond the scope of this book to address these issues, but we believe that participatory HF/E approaches have many strengths when it comes to engaging with under-represented groups, and this is what we will explore in this chapter. The chapter is based on guidance developed by the Chartered Institute of Ergonomics and Human Factors (CIEHF) (Grant, 2022).

This chapter might be of particular use for those involved in:

- Writing or updating organisational EDI strategies and related documentation
- Workforce planning
- Commissioning
- Service development

- Procurement
- Technology design
- Procedure development.

Why Are Many Health and Care Systems Not Inclusive?

The CIEHF guidance definitions of Equality, Diversity and Inclusion are provided in Table 10.1. The guidance summarises this as follows: 'equality is concerned with fairness, diversity is concerned with representation, and inclusion is concerned with involvement' (Grant, 2022). Implicit in this is the notion that health and care systems need to be actively designed to meet the needs of the system users, and, for this to happen, those users need to be involved in the co-design of these systems. If we return to the pandemic, we can see clear examples of care systems that were not designed to meet these needs. Early on, pulse oximetry became a key marker of acuity and was therefore used in triaging patients. Pulse oximetry is a non-invasive optical technique for measuring arterial oxygen saturation. Studies suggest that pulse oximetry is less accurate in patients with darker skin tones, and the effect is to over-estimate oxygen saturation, meaning that the severity of some patients' illness may not have been recognised (Al-Halawani et al., 2023; Cabanas et al., 2022). Furthermore, cutaneous presentations of COVID, such as rashes and the chilblain-like lesions associated with 'COVID toes', were also harder to see on darker skin. This was made worse by the lack of clinical images made available to allow healthcare professionals to understand what they were looking for. This also led to concerns that COVID was not being recognised quickly enough within groups that were known to have poorer outcomes (Akuffo-Addo et al., 2022).

TABLE 10.1 The meaning of the terms Equality, Diversity and Inclusion as described by Grant (2022)

Term	Meaning
Equality	**Equality** is about treating everyone fairly, regardless of the protected characteristics they hold. It is about ensuring everyone is given equal access to opportunities. It's closely related to **equity**, which is about addressing barriers that can prevent people from thriving and recognising that some people need more because they started with less.
Diversity	**Diversity** is about recognising people's differences. This includes both protected and non-protected characteristics. Considering diversity can mean explicitly monitoring the people's characteristics and identifying groups that are under-represented. Understanding the systemic reasons behind under-representation allows for positive action to address them.
Inclusion	**Inclusion** is about making sure everyone feels involved and that the environment they are in makes everyone as accepted and comfortable as each other. For example, the means of access to and within a space influences the extent to which the people using it can participate in activities. Ensuring inclusion might involve designing physical access to and within a space to allow everyone to easily access all areas.

Lack of inclusion continued to affect outcomes even in countries with excellent vaccine availability. Previous experiences of racism contributed to vaccine hesitancy and rendered many people vulnerable to disinformation (Peña et al., 2023). Even those who wished to be vaccinated struggled to access vaccination centres because of location, cost of travel, limited opening hours, reflecting the intersectionality described above (Kemei et al., 2023). Of course, it was not just race and ethnicity that were barriers to attending vaccination clinics – the design of vaccination centres (Sujan et al, 2021) often meant that people had to queue for long periods of time, with limited opportunities for sitting. Older people and those with co-morbidities often struggled.

While the pandemic brought some of these issues to the fore, it was only acting as a magnifying glass for problems that we already knew existed. For example, in the UK the national programme *Mothers and Babies: Reducing Risk through Audits and Confidential Enquiries across the UK* (MBRRACE-UK) highlighted ethnic and socioeconomic disparities in maternal and infant mortality rates. Box 10.1 contains a summary of some of the findings of the most recent MBRRACE-UK reports (Draper et al., 2023).

BOX 10.1 Examples of health disparities identified in the MBRRACE-UK reports

MBRRACE-UK is a UK-wide collaborative programme which forms part of one of the four Clinical Outcome Review Programmes overseen by the Healthcare Quality Improvement Partnership (HQIP) on behalf of the NHS organisations and governments of the UK. It aims to collect information about late fetal losses, stillbirths, neonatal and maternal deaths. MBRRACE was formed in 2013, but it is not entirely new: national confidential enquires into such events have been carried out every 20 years in the UK, driven by consistently high rates of perinatal mortality compared with other countries in Europe. MBRRACE still adopts the 'confidential enquiry' methodology. This means the data is extracted from what is available within the written documentation. This not only relies on accurate note taking, but also on the interpretation by staff of what is relevant for inclusion. It lacks much of the contextual information that is unlikely to have been captured in such documentation.

Cases are reviewed by a multi-disciplinary panel that includes representatives from all stages of the care pathway (for example, obstetricians, midwives, neonatologists and perinatal pathologists). Panels are selected to ensure appropriate ethnic representation. The aim is to consider each case and draw conclusions about the overall quality of care. If care was not of good quality, the enquiry seeks to establish whether this had an impact on outcomes.

The findings are relevant across the service but, as the reports show, outcomes are particularly poor for women and babies who are not White. For example, the most recent data suggests that Black women have a 124% increased risk of stillbirth and a 43% increase in risk of neonatal mortality when compared with White women.

Chapter 10 Equality, Diversity and Inclusion

> Examples of contributory factors include screening of Black women for gestational diabetes: often this was inconsistent and did not follow national guidelines. 30% of Black women who were eligible for an oral glucose tolerance test were not offered one, compared with 3% of White women. Similarly, if Black women are identified as being at risk of vitamin D deficiency, they need higher doses than White women. This is rarely recognised. Hypertension is a risk factor for stillbirth and neonatal death, but it was less likely to be picked up and treated in Black women. There were also differences in the way women and their families were treated after loss. It is considered good practice to address letters about follow-up appointments directly to the parents, rather than the GP. There is also guidance about how to write such letters in a clear and sensitive manner. It was less likely for Black women to receive a letter that followed this guidance.

The key findings of these reports can read like a long list of 'minor failings', but they speak to a wider issue that affects us all. Person-centred care and personalised care have become buzz words, but what does this mean in practice? It is a complex process of combining the generic and the specific: taking evidence-based guidelines that describe best practice for the general population, but trying to understand how these apply to the patient in front of you. This is difficult enough at the best of times, but what if those guidelines have been designed for a population that does not include the patient in front of you? Furthermore, what if there are significant cultural, social and economic differences that mean you cannot realistically understand that patient's perspective?

We are increasingly recognising that the design of many health and social care systems is based on principles that have their roots in colonialism, and therefore are largely best serving a White European population. For example, it has been suggested that even global health organisations are not truly global because the leadership positions are filled by more people who went to Harvard University than by women from developing countries (Abimola and Pai, 2020). Given that the majority of health and social care in such countries will be delivered by women, representation is not remotely adequate, and so the views, knowledge and skills of these frontline workers are not taken seriously. Even within some high-income countries, there is a problem of wealth distribution – they are often really just poor countries with a few very rich individuals. Trying to redesign health and social care to make them more inclusive is also likely to face challenge from those for whom it suits to maintain the status quo.

Protected Characteristics Are Person Factors

Protected characteristics are people factors, but ones which a country has chosen to protect by making it illegal to discriminate against. In the UK, EDI is governed by the Equality Act 2010, which recognises nine protected characteristics as shown in Figure 10.1.

Other countries, such as the US and Brazil, have similar legislation, and these legal responsibilities are often reflected in organisational documentation. Indeed,

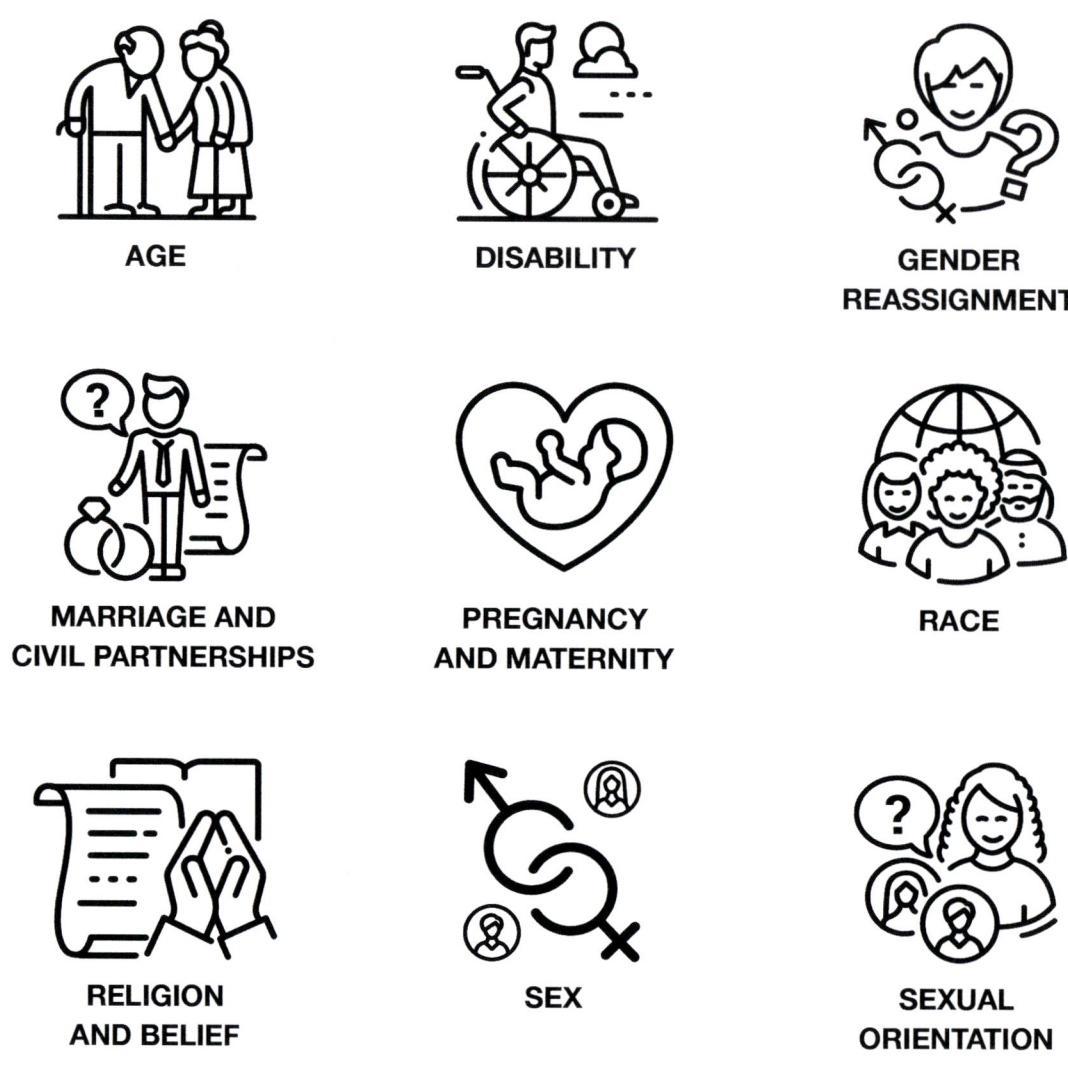

FIGURE 10.1 Protected characteristics in the UK.
Source: Grant, 2022.

it may well be that you are reading this chapter because you have been assigned responsibility for writing or updating your own organisational strategy or policies.

In addition to recognising these protected characteristics, it is important to remember that not all disabilities are obvious, and areas that are coming into increasing focus include things like neurodiversity and learning difficulties, such as dyslexia. Sensory deficits do not just involve blindness, but might also involve, for example, balance. We should also remember that deficits are not always permanent – some are caused by illness or injury of limited duration. This may be particularly relevant in countries where policy has moved towards 'fit notes' rather than 'sick notes'. The former capture details of the functional effects of a person's condition with a view to them being used as a basis for making adaptations that can allow a person to continue working. All of these need to be considered alongside social and economic factors.

Chapter 10   Equality, Diversity and Inclusion

Health and social care environments need to be designed to meet the needs of a broad range of diverse people and populations.

Given that we have already described protected characteristics (and others) as person factors, and mentioned the importance of context, it is not unreasonable to suggest that taking a systems approach is one of the most important things you can do to help address EDI issues. Before we do that, it is also worth considering what is often described in the literature as a relationship between protected characteristics and 'structural factors' (Flagg and Campbell, 2021). For example, if you are not White (in the UK) or are disabled, you are more likely to be out of work (or in low paid work), less likely to have a high educational achievement and less likely to live in accommodation that supports your needs (Otu et al., 2020, Maroto & Pettinicchio, 2014 and Aitken et al., 2018). Protected characteristics are, therefore, very much related to socioeconomic status, and therefore to health. From an HF/E perspective, we would consider 'structural' factors as system outcomes resulting from the interactions of different elements of the system.

Taking a Systems Approach to Highlight EDI Issues

To understand the impact that not considering EDI issues has on health and care system outcomes, it might be easier to start with the relatively simple example of prescribing. Healthcare professionals with prescribing responsibilities need to understand drug absorption, distribution, metabolism and excretion if they are to do so safely. If you are a prescriber, it is likely that your pharmacokinetics education began and ended in the patient's body. Indeed, that is often how we describe kinetics: 'what the body does to the drug.' However, people take medication within a system that extends far beyond that physical body. Taking a systems approach brings up relevant aspects that otherwise might not have been considered. In SEIPS (Systems Engineering Initiative for Patient Safety) terminology, absorption (the way in which drugs move from the site of administration into the bloodstream), distribution (how drugs move from the bloodstream to the tissues), metabolism (how drugs are chemically altered to facilitate their removal from the body) and excretion (the way in which drugs leave the body) can all be considered as processes. Outcomes include things like therapeutic response, but also adverse events etc. By viewing drug metabolism in this way, we can appreciate that it's often these wider systems factors that will determine how much drug is absorbed in the first place, how it is distributed and how it is ultimately removed from the body. A lack of consideration of these broader systems factors can often be seen to be behind many drug-related adverse events.

For example, consider insulin-dependent diabetes (Figure 10.2). A traditional approach might focus only on how insulin works in the body. A systems approach goes beyond this. Other outcomes, such as the impact that living with diabetes has on the ability to work and wider life circumstances, become important. People might have a fear of hypoglycaemic episodes (low blood sugar), and this might lead someone to reduce their insulin dose with negative consequences, or they might recognise that controlling the dose allows them to control their weight. In some cases, they may be unable to afford sufficient insulin in health systems where payment for medication is out of their own pocket. By examining these wider interactions, we can identify how social and economic factors can influence medication use and potentially worsen health outcomes for certain groups.

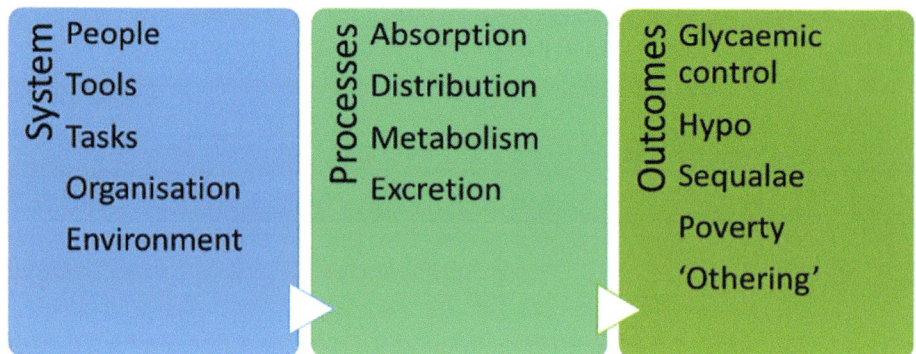

FIGURE 10.2 Systems perspective of insulin-dependent diabetes.

It is also worth remembering that these issues do not just apply to improving patient care, but equally apply to the experience of healthcare staff. If jobs, roles, physical environments, procedures and equipment, for instance, are not designed to account for the diversity of the workforce, then workers will be harmed by (and disadvantaged in) their jobs.

Participation as a Mechanism for Delivering Equality, Diversity and Inclusion

In the CIEHF EDI guidance, the systems approach is highlighted as a powerful tool for combating exclusion, especially when that exclusion is not conscious. It is also recognised that the systems approach is best for developing sustainable recommendations and solutions. In addition to this, the guidance makes the case for engaging with systems stakeholders to address EDI issues. However, it specifically highlights the importance of participatory HF/E. What does this mean? Surely all HF/E activity is participatory? We are aiming to engage with system stakeholders to understand their perspective, and they therefore participate in this activity! There is some truth in this, but the person leading the project and doing the systems analysis is making all the decisions: from identifying stakeholders and planning data collection, right through to making (and sometimes implementing) recommendations. Alternatively, it may be the case that the HF/E work is fed back to management, and they implement the findings. While these approaches are participatory to a certain extent, they are what Wilson (1995) described as 'consultative' or 'representative' participation. All of the activity will inevitably be shaped by the lens through which the HF/E lead (and the management) view the system.

'Direct' participation describes a different situation, where the system stakeholders (especially those at the sharp end) have a degree of power and influence when it comes to exploring work and making changes. The role of the project lead (and management) is a facilitatory one, co-ordinating activity and providing the necessary capital, whether that be power or another resource. It is viewed as a specific

Chapter 10 Equality, Diversity and Inclusion

BOX 10.2 Dimensions of a participatory conceptual framework (Haines et al., 2002)

- Location of decision-making power – whether retained by management and informed by consultation with individual workers or groups, or delegated to the workers.
- Mix of participants formed for the interventions – frontline staff only, or including technical staff, middle management and/or senior management.
- Remit – that is, the extent of the participants' involvement in setting up and monitoring of the participatory ergonomics process, the identification of problems to be addressed, and the generation, evaluation and implementation of solutions.
- Role of 'ergonomics specialist/s' – acknowledged as potentially changing and evolving over time, ranging from being a facilitator or leader, trainer, expert team member, or available for consultation as required (or not involved).
- Nature of worker involvement – varying from direct face-to-face involvement of all affected workers to representative participation of selected workers.
- Focus – whether aimed at the level of design of tasks undertaken by individuals or teams, or broader work organisation issues or policies.
- Level of influence – variations in the level of the organisation at which the intervention takes place, whether at the level of the work team or department, through to the entire organisation, or indeed, across an industry.
- Requirement – that is, whether the participation is undertaken by volunteers, or is an expected part of a job role, noting that this may vary across group members.
- Permanence of the intervention – ranging from a temporary programme introduced as means of solving a particular problem, to programmes intended to be permanently integrated into the ongoing continuous improvement activities of the organisation.

macro-ergonomic approach to the design of work, and Haines et al. (2002) proposed a conceptual framework. The dimensions of the framework are listed in Box 10.2. The order reflects the relative importance, as defined by Hignett et al. (2005). While the terminology all refers to 'workers', we can appreciate that the same principles could apply to engaging with patients and their families, and other service users.

Participatory ergonomics is not really a theory-driven concept, with a particular ascribed methodology. Its existence in the literature is almost the reverse: different researchers describe projects that have a participatory element to them, and retrospectively these have been grouped together under this name. What that means is the 'toolbox' for participatory approaches is very large and includes many of the methods we have covered in this book. Things such as systems frameworks, task analysis, interviews, focus groups, questionnaires, user testing, culture discussion cards, etc., can all be used as part of a participatory approach. Simulation, mock-ups, prioritised voting and problem-solving groups of various types are other tools to consider, and you can view an example later in this chapter.

What Might Participatory HF/E Look Like in Health and Social Care?

If participatory approaches are to be sustainable within organisations, we are really talking about establishing design processes in which end users can influence these processes, so they are compatible with their values, beliefs and desired outcomes. For this to be achievable, you can perhaps appreciate that there needs to be a depth and breadth of HF/E understanding across the organisation if systems stakeholders are to be able to participate in a meaningful way.

Figure 10.3 suggests that for HF/E approaches to be fully embedded across an organisation, everyone needs to have a basic awareness, while others within the organisation need to have a greater degree of expertise. Guidance can be provided by a much smaller number of suitably qualified and experienced experts. In many ways, this is the model this book is intended to support. It can be appreciated that, if a training element is embedded as part of the role of those staff with HF/E competence and experience, then there will be sufficient HF/E competence across the organisation to truly support a participatory approach.

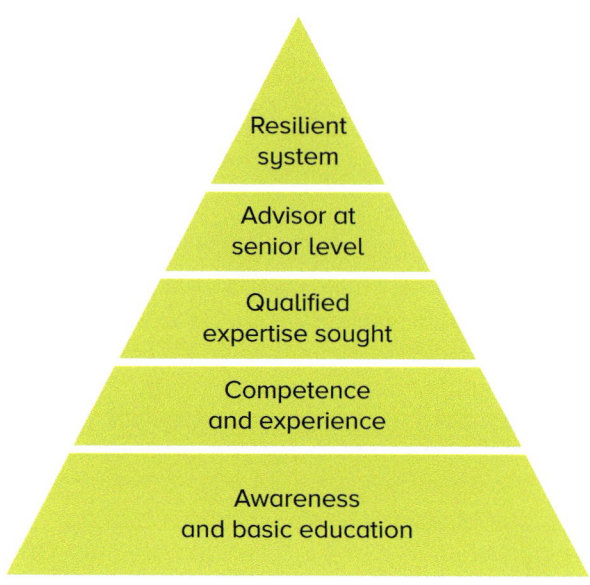

FIGURE 10.3 A vision for embedded HF/E competence across an organisation.

Source: The CIEHF White Paper for Health and Social Care, 2018.

ISO 27500 (The Human Centred Organization)

One option for organisations that are serious about addressing EDI is to consider adopting the principles described in the International Standard 27500 (International Organization for Standardization 2016). ISO 27500 is somewhat different from many other international standards – rather than complying with the standard, the intent is that organisations strive to live up to the principles. The main driver behind the development of the standard was recognition by G7 nations that human well-being is an important economic measure. The importance of well-being is currently being extensively discussed in many countries – pressures on health and social care staff have led to unsustainable recruitment and retention issues. ISO 27500 summarises the values and beliefs that make an organisation human-centred and suggests ways in which this may be achieved. ISO 27500 is underpinned by HF/E thinking, and there are seven defining principles (Table 10.2).

TABLE 10.2 Defining principles described in ISO 27500

No.	Principle
1.	Capitalise on individual differences as an organisational strength
2.	Make usability and accessibility strategic business objectives
3.	Adopt a total systems approach
4.	Ensure health, safety and well-being are business priorities
5.	Value employees and create a meaningful work environment
6.	Be open and trustworthy
7.	Act in socially responsible ways

ISO 27500 prioritises understanding of user needs and integrating HF/E thinking throughout the design, development, implementation, and maintenance of processes and systems (Principle 1). This includes designing systems that are easy to learn, use and maintain, considering people's needs and their experience (Principle 2). The standard also encourages a culture that values safety, openness and transparency, and learning from events (Principle 3). It emphasises designing meaningful work that contributes to a broader range of outcomes, which include human well-being, encompassing both physical and mental health (Principles 4 and 5). ISO 27500 promotes continuous improvement based on data, feedback and evolving needs, while valuing user (patient, families and carers in a health and social care context) and staff participation and expertise throughout these activities (Principles 6 and 7).

Case Study: Participatory Design of a Neonatal Resuscitation Monitoring Device

Embarking on a study to understand the needs and requirements of healthcare staff in monitoring neonatal resuscitation required consideration of the inclusion of the whole team. The differences across roles and experience were considered in obtaining a representative sample of stakeholders. This ensured inclusion of both novices and experts, the leaders and professional roles typically adopted in this time-critical and emergency situation. The emotive nature of the situation was also considered. Ideally those with lived experience would have been included, but the risk of re-traumatising families was considered too great to justify their inclusion. The study adopted a participatory approach to produce essential and desirable design requirements for a medical device interface, which aimed to improve the ease and reliability of monitoring neonatal heart rate (Pickup et al., 2019).

A user-centred design method was used, the Applied Cognitive Task Analysis (ACTA) (Militello and Hutton, 1998); see also Chapter 3 for a reminder of task analysis methods. This method supports the extraction of knowledge around the decision making and cognitive requirements for the clinician in dealing with this scenario, while also seeking to understand the potential errors for both experts and novices.

The output from this initial method informed a workshop involving all relevant job roles. The workshop included a low-fidelity simulation of a neonatal resuscitation, with a focus on the key decision-making and cognitive tasks, perceived as critical to the interface design. There were several resources required to ensure the success of the workshop: pens, paper, cardboard boxes and pizza! The last item set the tone of the workshop, reinforcing the message this was not about assessing competence, and thanking staff for their knowledge and expertise.

Cardboard boxes were used to capture the intended interface design and highlight the basic (essential) and future (desirable) properties of the interface. This was achieved by simply drawing onto a blank box that acted as the intended new device in the scenario (Figure 10.4). Group discussions were facilitated, and two mock-ups of potential interfaces were produced. Staff were encouraged to discuss the reasoning behind their designs, and then each participant was given the opportunity to

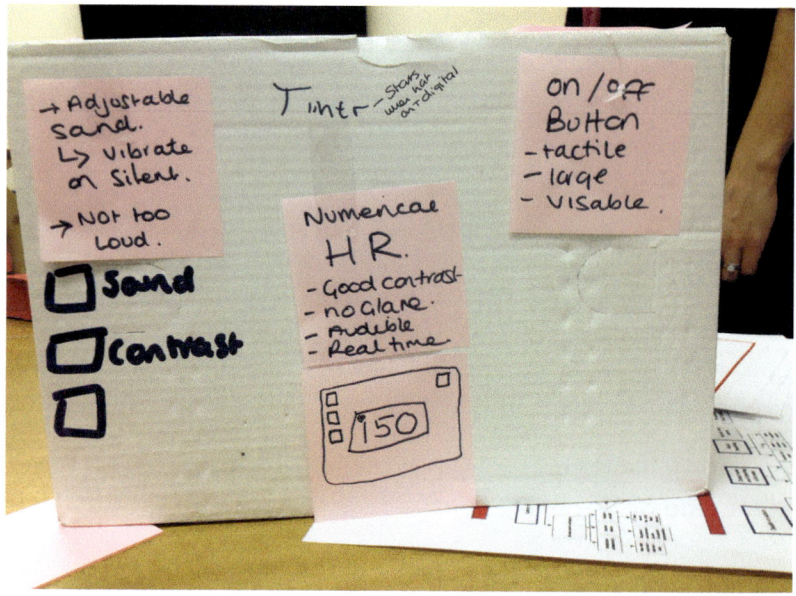

FIGURE 10.4 Cardboard boxing to support intended user interface design.

Source: © Laura Pickup.

independently draw their personal preference for the design. The analysis following the workshop produced a heat map to illustrate a general consensus of where key displays and controls should be located on the future interface.

Adopting a participatory approach ensured engagement of the whole group in specifying the core design requirements. The use of cardboard boxes and simple props enabled inclusion of all participants to engage and demonstrate their thoughts captured in a simple but effective way. The outputs from this work included: a high-level representation of neonatal resuscitation tasks; identification of the cognitive requirements for key tasks, critical information and decision points; analysis of the cognitive demands and potential errors. Participants reflected that the approach provided a systematic way to understand and justify the final interface design. The workshop produced novel factors that were not previously recognised and were included in the final design, which is now commercially available.

Chapter Summary

This chapter introduced basic considerations relating to equality, diversity and inclusion. The key message is that taking a participatory ergonomics approach can be a powerful means of identifying and capturing the voices of those who are often not represented in our improvement activity. It is true that participatory approaches are challenging. They require empowering, resourcing and supporting participants to actively drive change. Clearly, this is not something that can be achieved without organisational commitment. It would be worth considering this chapter alongside any plan for human factors integration (Chapter 11).

CIEHF HF/E Competencies

Use of a human-centred approach to the design and development of systems
- Understands the role and application of HF/E principles in optimising system performance and well-being across all ages and capabilities.
- Demonstrates ability to enhance health, safety, comfort, quality of life, attitudes, motivation, usability, effectiveness and efficiency.

Focus on how other system components and performance-influencing factors affect people
- Determines the match and the interaction between human characteristics, abilities, capacities and motivations, and the system(s), organisation, planned or existing environment, products used, equipment, work systems, machines and tasks.

Professional skills and behaviours
- Understands role of HF/E in change strategies.

References

Abimbola, S. & Pai, M. 2020. Will global health survive its decolonisation? *The Lancet*, 396(10263), 1627–1628.

Aitken, Z., Baker, E., Badland, H., et al. 2018. Precariously placed: Housing affordability, quality and satisfaction of Australians with disabilities. *Disability & Society*, 34(1), 121–142.

Akuffo-Addo, E., Nicholas, M. N. & Joseph, M. 2022. COVID-19 skin manifestations in skin of colour. *Journal of Cutaneous Medicine and Surgery*, 26(2), 189–197.

Al-Halawani, R., Charlton, P. H., Qassem, M., et al. 2023. A review of the effect of skin pigmentation on pulse oximeter accuracy. *Physiological Measurement*, 44(5), 05TR01.

Cabanas A. M., Fuentes-Guajardo, M., Latorre, K., et al. 2022. Skin pigmentation influence on pulse oximetry accuracy: A systematic review and bibliometric analysis. *Sensors*, 22(9), 3402.

Chartered Institute for Ergonomics and Human Factors. 2018. *White Paper for Health and Social Care. A vision for integrating Human Factors in Health and Social Care*. Chartered Institute of Ergonomics and Human Factors.

Draper E.S., Gallimore I.D., Kurinczuk J.J., et al, (eds.), on behalf of the MBRRACE-UK Collaboration. 2023. MBRRACE-UK Perinatal Confidential Enquiry, A comparison of the care of Black and White women who have experienced a stillbirth or neonatal death: State of the Nation Report. Leicester: The Infant Mortality and Morbidity Studies, Department of Population Health Sciences, University of Leicester.

Flagg, L.D. & Campbell, L.A. 2021. COVID-19 in Communities of Color: Structural Racism and Social Determinants of Health. *Online Journal of Issues in Nursing*, 26(2), 1–11.

Fouad, M. N., Ruffin, J. & Vickers, S. M. 2020. COVID-19 is disproportionately high in African Americans. This will come as no surprise… . *American Journal of Medicine*, 133(10), e544–e545.

Grant, C. 2022. *How human factors can enhance the delivery of equality, diversity and inclusion (EDI)*. Chartered Institute of Ergonomics and Human Factors.

Haines, H., Wilson, J.R., Vink, P., et al. 2002. Validating a framework for participatory ergonomics (the PEF). *Ergonomics* 45, 309–327.

Hignett, S., Wilson, J.R. & Morris, W. 2005. Finding ergonomic solutions—participatory Approaches. *Occupational Medicine* 55:200–207.

International Organization for Standardization. 2016. *The human-centred organization — Rationale and general principles*. https://www.iso.org/obp/ui/#iso:std:iso:27500:ed-1:v1:en

Kemei, J., Tulli, M., Olanlesi-Aliu, A., et al. 2023. Impact of the COVID-19 pandemic on Black communities in Canada. *International Journal of Environmental Research and Public Health*, 20(2), 1580.

Maroto, M., & Pettinicchio, D. 2014. Disability, structural inequality, and work: The influence of occupational segregation on earnings for people with different disabilities. *Research in Social Stratification and Mobility*, 38, 76–92.

Mathieu, E., Ritchie, H., Rodés-Guirao, L., et al. 2020. Coronavirus Disease (COVID-19). *Our World in Data*, 1(1). https://ourworldindata.org/coronavirus

Militello, L.G. & Hutton, R.J.B. 1998. Applied cognitive task analysis (ACTA): a practitioner's toolkit for understanding cognitive task demands. *Ergonomics*, 41(11), 1618–1641.

Otu, A., Ahinkorah, B. O., Ameyaw, E. K., et al. 2020. One country, two crises: What COVID-19 reveals about health inequalities among BAME communities in the United Kingdom and the sustainability of its health system. *International Journal for Equity in Health*, 19(1), 189.

Peña, J. M., Schwartz, M. R., Hernandez-Vallant, A., et al. 2023. Social and structural determinants of COVID-19 vaccine uptake among racial and ethnic groups. *Journal of Behavioral Medicine*, 46, 129–139.

Pickup L., Lang A., Shipley L., et al. 2019. Development of a Clinical Interface for a Novel Newborn Resuscitation Device: Human Factors Approach to Understanding Cognitive User Requirements. *JMIR Human Factors* 6(2):e12055

Sujan, M., Hignett, S. & Rashid, N. 2021. *Vaccinating a nation: Ten human factors and ergonomics principles*. Chartered Institute of Ergonomics and Human Factors.

WHO. 2020. *A global pandemic requires a world effort to end it – none of us will be safe until everyone is safe*. https://www.who.int/news-room/commentaries/detail/a-global-pandemic-requires-a-world-effort-to-end-it-none-of-us-will-be-safe-until-everyone-is-safe

Wilson, J. R. 1995. Ergonomics and participation. In: Wilson, J. R. & Corlett, E. N. (eds.), *Evaluation of human work: A practical ergonomics methodology, Second Edition*. Taylor and Francis.

CHAPTER 11

Human Factors Integration

Chapter Objectives and Learning Outcomes

- To understand the term and the approach of human factors integration.
- To distinguish the difference between human factors integration as a management process and the science underpinning human factors and ergonomics.
- To understand the justification for and core components of human factors integration.
- To consider the opportunities and application of human factors integration into health and social care.

Introduction: Developing Processes for Embedding and Evidencing Human Factors/Ergonomics

Implementation of health and social care work and technical systems needs to optimise the needs, capability and experience of those required to deliver and receive these services. To achieve this, it is essential to fully understand the role, requirements, needs and capabilities of people, and to fully integrate these properties with the equipment and systems developed and provided by health and social care services. Integration is the best approach to optimising the capability and experience of real-world care settings. Human factors integration (HFI) is the approach adopted in other safety-critical industries to ensure human needs and capabilities are considered, and people are effectively integrated into equipment and system design, procurement and implementation. HF/E is a broad discipline, and health and social care is yet to fully apply HF/E to support all domains or goals intended to improve services and patient safety.

There are two international standards that are helpful to consider and that place people at the centre of organisational goals: 'The Human Centred Organization – rationale and general principles' (ISO 27500:2016(E)) and 'The design of system and equipment – Ergonomics of human-system interaction – Part 210: Human-centred design for interactive systems' (ISO 9241-210:2010). These could be useful resources to support health and social care to integrate with the human-centred systems approach applied by HFI.

This chapter will consider the core characteristics of HFI providing some insight to the background and approach, as well as where health and social care could benefit from HFI, the potential challenges faced, and suggestions for practical opportunities to embed this approach to meet existing health and social care needs.

This chapter might be of particular use for:

- Professionals adopting a leading role in human factors for a health or social care organisation.
- Managers and leaders interested in developing human factors to support safety, performance and well-being.
- The development, procurement and implementation of services and equipment.
- Risk and governance teams considering the management and mitigation of organisational risks.
- Digital leads and clinical engineering teams.

Human Factors Integration Principles

Human factors integration refers to the management and systematic process adopted for recognising, evaluating, monitoring and addressing hazards and issues relating to the interaction of humans with the technical systems employed (traditionally), as well as with the other elements of a work system, such as the physical environment. This is different from HF/E, which refers to the science and evidence applied to understand and inform system, process and equipment design.

HFI aims to equally consider and optimise technical and human capabilities to achieve an organisation's goals. There is a long history in other industries of recognising that failure to consider human needs and capabilities in the original design or implementation of technical and work systems has a number of undesirable consequences, which include increased time and cost for redesign, higher cost for training, increased frequency of incidents and time required to investigate them, reduced performance and efficiencies, and loss of skilled staff. The efficiency of an entire system will always be dependent upon how well the design has considered the interaction of the human, their needs and capabilities, with all other elements of the system, such as environment, technology and equipment, and tasks. A human-centred design (ISO 9241-210:2010) approach describes how an organisation can deliver the economic and social value of a system, while ensuring they also meet safety requirements and avoid harm to those delivering, using or experiencing the system.

The military and the railway industry have good examples of guidance that support the expectation of HFI to exist in the introduction or design of a new system, with clear categories to be considered throughout any project. Their guidance mirrors a human-centred design approach, and both are publicly available and are recommended reading to further explain what HFI practically looks like (Ministry of Defence Parts 1 and 2, 2021; Office of Rail and Road, 2016). The military suggests a

Chapter 11 Human Factors Integration

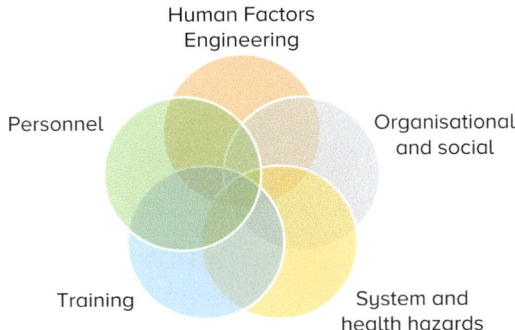

FIGURE 11.1 The five domains of HFI used in the military.

framework for HFI, which includes five domains to focus on, where HF/E work should be directed and established (Figure 11.1).

1. Personnel – how many people, the training required and the physical and cognitive requirements to operate and maintain the work system, in normal, degraded and emergency contexts.
2. Training – what is required to ensure the knowledge and skills to operate and maintain a system from an individual to a team perspective. This stresses the value of effectiveness of training to build team cohesion, tests of team structures and standard operating procedures.
3. Human factors engineering – the design and development of the system to integrate knowledge of human physical and cognitive capabilities. This requires analysis, such as task analysis, heuristics and interface analysis, workload analysis, postural, layout and environment analysis, to inform specifications for design and evaluation of new or existing solutions. This aims to ensure development of usable, safe and maintainable solutions to perform in all contexts.
4. System safety and health hazards – consideration of the potential risk to people or the system when working in normal and degraded contexts. Anticipate potential harm either to people using or working within the system – for example, musculoskeletal harm, mental health, spread of infection – as well as harm to equipment or physical environments and the likelihood of the error.
5. Organisational and social – recognising and understanding organisational behaviour and cultures through knowledge of organisational psychology, social science and management studies. Recognising organisational design and goals will influence performance and behaviours.

The guidance offered by the Office of Rail and Road outlines the objectives, a set of principles to be met and the evidence the regulator will look for to ensure HFI has met their standards (ORR, 2016). This provides a requirement for the Rail industry to embed and apply HF/E knowledge at all stages of a project and to the management of risk. The regulatory support and formal guidance to HFI has supported the established approach and employment of HF/E expertise across these industries.

Currently, within health and social care this level of guidance or expectation does not exist. However, this can be aspired to even at a local level within the health and social care environments we become involved with.

Why is Human Factors Integration Necessary for Health and Social Care?

In 2018, CIEHF, as the UK professional body for HF/E, published a White paper (CIEHF, 2018) to describe the aspiration for HF/E to be integrated within health and social care. This document recognised how other industries had achieved integration and outlined a vision for HF/E implementation in health and social care to include the following statements:

1. HF/E good practice is common across all health and social care processes, including audit, new and redesigned services, investigation and procurement.
2. HF/E is integrated across local, regional and national health and social care within all sectors of care.
3. The application of proven strategies for HF/E implementation with sector-specific competence frameworks.
4. International standards for HF/E are embedded within design and systems for planning and managing safety.
5. The underlying culture is a learning culture and an aspiration to improve human performance and well-being.

Fundamentally, the integration of HF/E ensures the sustainability of an organisation to embed HF/E, but also the effectiveness HF/E can have in systematically supporting the identification and management of emerging and existing risks. Small demonstrations of HF/E in single areas of care or design of services can be necessary to provide evidence and to model what HF/E can offer. However, without clarity in processes and a strategy to embed HF/E within existing health and social care processes, the potential for HF/E applications may not be realised.

In health and social care, we don't have to look hard for examples within our organisations of technical systems that have been procured but may not achieve their intended purpose – or may even make it harder for staff to complete their work reliably and confidently. This may also be true of new processes, which are introduced to achieve a goal of greater efficiency or even safety, but increase the workload or rely on increased staff capabilities to be effective. The term 'unintended consequences' can often be overused, and perhaps we need to consider in some cases that it may be more a case of 'unconsidered consequences', if we cannot demonstrate a process that seeks to anticipate the systemic impact of a project or product related to people. HFI is the process that can enable this in the early stages of a project or procurement process and can support identifying potential risks or unintended consequences.

The example given in Box 11.1 is hypothetical; however, it echoes several issues observed by the authors in their own practice. Technology intended to provide a

Chapter 11 Human Factors Integration

BOX 11.1 Illustration of how HFI can improve system design

> Let us assume an organisation relies on the data collected through incident reports to learn about issues experienced by staff and patients. They might consider the technical system implemented an effective way to collect this data on a day-to-day basis. On collating and analysing the data, they might identify human error as the cause for poor data entry and categorisation of incidents. However, such a conclusion might not consider the usability of the interface design and a system that staff may need to access during high caseloads or at the end of a twelve-hour shift, where fatigue and the need to rest before the next shift is also a priority.
>
> HFI would enable early consideration and a systematic approach to the system and human requirements to inform a user-centred design approach to incident reporting systems. A user-centred approach would engage relevant stakeholders and understand user requirements and the context of reporting. The application of HF/E knowledge on interface design to support usability of the system at the design stage, and recognition of likely use errors, can inform how input and output data may be compromised through different design options. HFI is the process that would ensure evaluation, testing and an iterative approach to the design process to consider people, system requirements to increase reliability in the breadth of work contexts and organisational behaviours and culture that may challenge the collection of incident data collection. The depth of insight gained through HFI enhances the usability of systems and minimises training requirements, as well as cost spent on redesign.

safety-critical or learning and reporting function may be poorly designed, without consideration of the diversity of users, their needs and requirements, or the intended function of the system.

There are different stages to integration, and the maturity of an organisation's approach to HF/E can provide a useful benchmarking exercise. The maturity scale in Figure 11.2 offers some goals to describe the implementation journey (Edmonds and Gray, 2019).

An organisation with an HFI strategy would enable HF/E methods and principles to be implemented into organisational procurement and redesign processes, and these processes would enable the development or design of work systems that are based on realistic human capabilities. An HFI strategy ensures HF/E knowledge becomes integral to the organisational culture and is consistently applied to support the practice of designing safety into systems, work processes and technology.

What Could Human Factors Integration Look Like in Health and Social Care?

Despite the generic term of health and social care, we do not find the same organisational structures across the same type of provider. For example, the

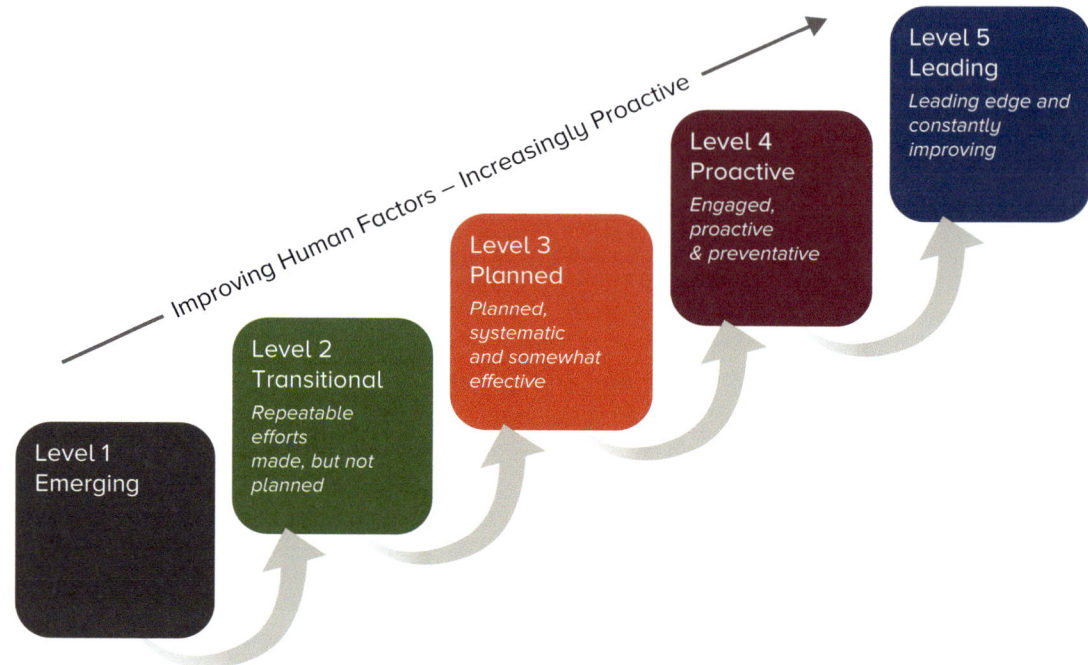

FIGURE 11.2 Human Factors Integration (HFI) Maturity Scale.
Source: Edmonds and Gray, 2019.

division of specialties may vary and the corporate structure and grouping of certain organisational functions, such as governance, safety, improvement and procurement, may look distinctly different between organisations. This means that HFI needs to understand these different organisational structures to fully consider how and where human factors expertise is needed, and where best to place leadership around the co-ordination of human factors resources.

Traditionally in healthcare, silos are recognised as challenging to clinical work and the implementation of change and improvements. The division of departments and expertise may stem from organisational history or perhaps a desire to manage a very large system by decomposition and simplification of the component parts (Hollnagel, 2021). It may be unintended, but the consequence is that a chasm can develop between expertise and potential learning from these different areas.

Silos in workstreams are created as some in the organisation drive a focus specifically in one direction, perhaps to improve quality and staff well-being, while others consider performance and safety. This differentiation may create a lack of visibility in the association of staff safety metrics and patient safety metrics, preventing the identification of signals that may indicate an interdependency between the two. Such divisions can also challenge the integration of human factors with the principle of considering and optimising safety, well-being and performance for people and the organisation. Co-ordinating efforts across these different divisions is required by human factors practitioners in health and social care. This requires a need for skills that are familiar to any human factors practitioner, which include the ability to communicate and explain how and why HFI is of value, while avoiding being perceived as a threat to familiar, established and relied-upon practices. Change takes time, and HFI is a change that healthcare is increasingly showing an appetite for; however, confidence in what and how this looks is yet to be achieved. Demonstration of HF/E in practice is essential to showcase how adopting a systems approach can support or contribute alongside other disciplines.

The development of an approach to capture what HF/E looks likes and the delivery of case studies to key organisational roles is essential. This should aim to provide a realistic view of how HFI can be achieved on a small scale, to develop the motivation to upscale efforts. These key roles will inevitably have greater knowledge than the HF/E expert in how to make it happen. In the authors' experience the level of HF/E education in health and social care has grown significantly in the past ten years. In the context of a healthcare organisation, there may be many staff that have taken an interest and attended or completed different levels of HF/E courses or qualifications. Taking time to identify these individuals and understand the quality of knowledge across an organisation could be one way to swell knowledge and expertise available to an organisation. Those with roles in simulation, medicine management, critical or emergency care, anaesthesia and manual handling or health and safety appear to have been early adopters of available HF/E education. There are also many other roles that will include staff with expertise aligned with HF/E, including clinical engineers, equipment procurement teams and professionals working within risk teams and psychology, occupational health and well-being teams. Seeking common ground and existing expertise may provide opportunities to integrate HF/E with less difficulty. As a note of caution, seek to clarify whether your version of HF/E as a systems approach is the same as those working in different areas, as sometimes the core principles of HF/E can be lost in translation, and the practice of HF/E frequently is unduly limited to a narrow set of interventions around non-technical skills and teamwork. Finally, without a champion for HF/E at a senior level of the organisation, far-reaching integration will remain an uphill struggle. Therefore, focusing on the the completion of smaller-scale HF/E pieces of work may provide greater job satisfaction. This may still have a positive impact for local healthcare teams and even encourage senior leaders to become a HF/E champion.

What Might We Need to Consider to Develop a Human Factors Integration Strategy?

In every industry the structure and culture will play a significant part in what HFI might look like, but also in how it can be achieved. Leadership in integration may fall to an HF/E professional known to the organisation, or a completely new HF/E role may be developed. There are pros and cons to both of these scenarios; however, it is critical that either context recognises that 'what to do' and 'how to get it done' are equally relevant to the likely success of the implementation. The inter-relationships between HF/E practitioners and those who control existing organisational procedures or processes are critical. In healthcare, this may include clinical leads, improvement teams, teams responsible for the infrastructure and procurement, health and safety, patient safety and risk and governance teams. Here, existing relationships may support or increase the trust in the HF/E professional, while, equally, historic work practices and the silos recognised above can hinder embedding HF/E as a discipline that will seek to bridge teams that structurally may separate safety, performance and well-being. A new HF/E role or new face can provide opportunities for new ways of thinking, but finding whom to engage with and limiting fears or threats of an HF/E invasion may be the challenge. An established figure within an organisation may hold tacit knowledge, yet may also never shake perceptions held of their previous role. An expert by experience, Barry Kirwan shares his valuable lessons for HF/E professionals to take heed of the need to develop relationships and address organisational problems or goals rather than overwhelm people with HF/E principles and methods (Kirwan, 2000). Kirwan stresses the need to work in hybrid teams to gain trust and insight on how HF/E can contribute, and when it can be of greatest value. He cautions that sometimes HF/E practitioners may focus on the technical perspective in the application of certain methods when, ultimately, the organisation will take greater notice if a practical problem is improved.

Considering the softer side of the system you find yourself in is critical to understanding the best approach for developing an integration strategy. Ideally, we would consider HF/E to have a role across departments influential to safety and risks inherent to the organisation, operational processes that rely on humans for their safety or performance and finally in the context of the design of new infrastructure, technical and manual systems. Preferably, HF/E is recognised in organisational policies to ensure early engagement of HF/E in the project management plan; this may reduce the likelihood of HF/E being perceived as the messenger of bad news and the cause of delays to implementation, with suggestions for the need to redesign to address safety concerns.

This final section provides early thoughts on how to build HF/E capacity within health and social care organisations delivering services and care. Table 11.1 highlights examples of focused elements from a systems perspective that an organisation could consider HF/E to be actively engaged in. This is by no means an exhaustive list but seeks to demonstrate how HF/E can stretch across existing organisational structures and processes rather than focus purely on behavioural change of staff, which is traditionally how HF/E has been applied in healthcare. These include elements that are also recognised in the literature as HF/E elements that have been identified across industries and contributory to major accidents (Edmonds and Gray, 2019).

How to deliver HF/E to an organisation will again depend upon the organisation's size and function; one size will not fit all. Having a high level of expertise to facilitate and guide organisations, while also identifying or developing greater HF/E capacity, may lend itself to a 'hub and spoke' model. The hub of the HF/E provision would hold the highest level of HF/E qualification or expertise, extending its reach to individuals placed throughout the organisation. This could support broad engagement and specific HF/E knowledge relevant to an organisation's function. For example, knowledge of user-centred design and usability testing may significantly inform digital safety and implementation teams. Not everyone needs to be an expert in all areas of HF/E. However, there is a need for a basic level of knowledge on HF/E principles and some

TABLE 11.1 Human Factors elements influential to organisational safety, performance and well-being

Organisation	Tasks	People	Environment	Tools and technology	Measurement and system learning
Safety culture	Task performance	Human performance	Hazard identification	Procurement	System performance
Organisational culture	Everyday work and system analysis	Physical capabilities	Layout and design	Principles of good design	Well-being
Organisational change	Failure analysis	Cognitive capabilities	Performance-influencing factors: noise, light, temperature	Evaluating design	System safety
Organisational learning	Risk analysis	Performance-influencing factors	Health and well-being	Inclusive design	Reporting systems
Policies and procedures		User requirements/needs/accessibility		Implementation	Incident investigation
Work design		User-centred and participatory design			User experience
Management of safety		Non-technical skills			
Management of well-being		Teams – work, decision making and training			
Education					

basic tools to support local issues. Recognising the resource available, the opportunity to upskill staff or develop in-house training can be understood once the intended HF/E support structure is designed and a training-needs analysis can be created.

Coming back to the human factors maturity model presented earlier in the chapter (see Figure 11.2), this could be used to benchmark the current level of HF/E integration an organisation can evidence. Considering the different elements of HF/E, which are illustrated in Table 11.1, organisations can, as a group of representative stakeholders, grade the current level of maturity for each element. This would require descriptors at each level of the maturity scale to provide examples of what should be in place. This exercise is intended to benchmark and continue to evaluate organisational integration of HF based on what is actually in place rather than the perceptions of stakeholders (Edmonds and Gray, 2019).

This approach could be useful to develop a shared language across the breadth of HF/E elements, while offering an opportunity to demonstrate impact if HF/E is embedded. There may also be the need to increase knowledge and understanding of why integration of HF/E may benefit an organisation; this form of presentation can structure the discussion around organisational requirements and opportunities. Finally, it may also provide the opportunity to bring different parts of an organisation together, to break down the silos that may exist which have the potential to act as a barrier to HFI.

Chapter Summary

In this chapter you have been introduced to the concept of human factors integration (HFI). Examples have been provided of HFI in the context of other industries to share how this has been achieved and where they have focused their resources. The chapter makes the case for health and social care to consider what HFI could look like to enable a more sustainable and effective approach to delivering HF in line with existing organisational structures and goals. This chapter will enable you to reflect on how this may look in your organisation and invites you to design your own HFI strategy.

CIEHF HF/E Competencies

Use of a human-centred approach to the design and development of systems
- Understands the role and application of HF/E principles in optimising system performance and well-being across all ages and capabilities.

Professional skills and behaviours
- Understands role of HF/E in change strategies.
- Develops appropriate recommendations for education and training in relation to HF/E principles.

References

CIEHF. 2018. *Human Factors in Health & Social Care. White Paper*. https://ergonomics.org.uk/resource/human-factors-in-health-and-social-care.html

Edmonds, J. & Gray, K. 2019. Assessing human factors maturity. *Chemical Engineering Transactions*, 77, 481–486.

Hollnagel, E. 2021. *Synesis: The unification of productivity, quality, safety and reliability*. Routledge.

Kirwan, B. 2000. Soft systems, hard lessons. *Applied Ergonomics*, 31, 663–678.

Ministry of Defence. 2021. *JSP 912: Human Factors Integration for defence systems (Part 1: Directive)*. Ministry of Defence.

Ministry of Defence. 2021. *JSP 912: Human Factors Integration for defence systems (Part 2: Guidance)*. Ministry of Defence.

Office of Rail and Road (ORR). 2016. *Human factors integration – Objectives, principles and evidence ORR looks for*. https://www.orr.gov.uk/media/15720.

CHAPTER 12
Epilogue: The Future of Human Factors/Ergonomics in Health and Social Care

Introduction

The aim of this book is to inform and inspire those looking to apply HF/E principles to understand and improve health and social care. Structuring chapters around a systems engineering framework emphasises the 'systems thinking' that is a core foundation for HF/E. Human factors is not just concerned with the 'factors of the human', but with how humans interact with their wider context. Behaviours, both desirable and undesirable, are shaped by the skills and intent of the individual, the tasks they are required to perform, the technologies and tools available to them, their working environment, and its organisational, political and social structure and history. While we hope that this has provided a wealth of practical insights and approaches, there is no single formula, manual or recipe for HF/E. The professional application benefits from a broad set of analytical approaches, their skilled application, creativity and the building of relationships that allow the implementation and delivery of HF/E methods, analysis and work designs.

In the context of health and social care, HF/E considerations often stretch across organisational silos and boundaries. Different departments are separated with intentions of providing a focus on separate functions, yet they can profoundly affect one another in many ways. Well-facilitated HF/E can bring different departments together, providing opportunities to recognise and balance priorities across departments. However, this may also challenge traditional approaches to improvement, which often seek to fix problems locally without recognising wider influences. Sensitivity and a well-practised explanation of what HF/E is and how it approaches system change may reassure and promote collaborations, while also supporting the integration of HF/E into an organisation's existing practices. An elevator pitch about HF/E and why and how it works can be extremely helpful to rehearse.

It is important to recognise that HF/E is fundamentally a design discipline. Practitioners seek to understand and improve the complex interactions that contribute to the safety, well-being and performance of people and organisations. The reality of health and social care work systems is that they are messy. Variability is not just the norm but may be an essential characteristic to the success of many services. Adaptations and workarounds are necessary to deliver everyday care. Safety is an emergent organisational outcome, influenced by people, but dependent upon so much more. We rely on people to hold the system together, by recognising and mitigating risks, balancing conflicting outcomes and supporting each other. While we can certainly train behaviours such as teamwork and hazard awareness, this alone will fail to deliver the sustainable improvements essential for cultural change and safety. This book offers methods that support the representation of these systems to help to understand safety, inform improvement and design sustainable change.

There remains a need to weave HF/E principles throughout the structures and organisational functions that influence the safety, performance and well-being of people. Realisation of the full benefits of HF/E beyond relatively simple opportunistic projects requires a much longer-term strategy. Individual health and social care organisations require a senior leadership who will champion HF/E to become embedded into the organisation as part of the 'usual' business. We must also grow the capacity to provide experienced HF/E professionals in health and social care, working to provide the regulatory and professional support that can drive the application of HF/E to the level that is needed. The aspiration is that HF/E in health and social care could eventually come to resemble best practice in other industries, where HF/E informs policies, acquisition of equipment or infrastructure and processes that balance the need for performance with safety and well-being.

The Evolving Landscape of Health and Social Care

Health and social care have to cope with significant pressures, demographic changes and the development of disruptive technologies, including artificial intelligence (AI). It is worth considering how such trends and changes in health and social care will affect the application of HF/E, and where the approaches illustrated in this book might inform and influence these possible futures.

Technological innovation remains a cornerstone of sustainable change. It is certain to affect health and social care in an inconceivable number of ways. The use of AI, in particular, inspires hope for faster, cheaper and more personalised care, while at the same time fuelling fears of job losses, dehumanised medicine, and even greater health disparities as existing biases are reinforced. Back in 2016, Geoffrey Hinton, a Turing Award winner and 2024 Nobel Prize in Physics recipient for his contribution to the development of deep learning, famously declared that we should stop training radiologists because *it was obvious* that within five years deep learning was going to do better than radiologists. Eight years on we are starting to see the first dents in this AI hype and maybe a sense of reality setting in. Hinton has since qualified his claim, actual success stories of healthcare AI in use have been thin on the ground, and radiologists are, arguably, in greater demand than ever given the major diagnostic backlog both within the NHS and worldwide.

We still see frequent headlines that herald a new age of AI and autonomous healthcare practice, for example the story of the Smart Tissue Autonomous Robot (STAR), which performed surgery on pigs without human intervention. Increasingly, however, such headlines are accompanied by critical review that challenges the

Chapter 12   Epilogue

simplistic, technology-centric assumption that AI technologies might simply substitute for and improve on tasks previously done by people. Technology developers and healthcare providers are starting to recognise that the introduction of AI changes the way people work and how healthcare processes are delivered and managed.

Applications of AI require integration into existing care systems, and will need to be designed, operated and maintained by humans at some level. Some will have profound and lasting impacts on patients, clinicians and care systems. Others will be less successful. Some may prove to be dangerous. Considering the implications for human use within the system will help to ensure better designs, training, integration and evaluation. It may also help predict likely successes and failures. Involving HF/E practitioners – both those working to design technologies, and those working with clinicians at the front lines of care – offers both financial, safety and operational benefits. Ideally HF/E considerations should start early in the conception and design process, continuing through the verification, evaluation, widespread application and ongoing performance monitoring. In 2021, the Chartered Institute of Ergonomics and Human Factors (CIEHF) published the White Paper on *Human Factors and Ergonomics in Healthcare AI* in collaboration with both national and international partners, which formulated principles for designing healthcare AI (CIEHF, 2021). It is hoped that these principles will help future stakeholders move beyond focusing solely on the AI technology itself and instead take a human-centred, system perspective.

There will be significant shifts in demographics with an increasingly ageing population. The consequences of globalisation in general, and climate change in particular, are also likely to bring increases in migration and cultural diversity. The characteristics of the humans delivering and receiving care are therefore almost certain to change. Helping patients to live longer at home, delivering more care remotely in non-clinical environments, and learning to deal with compounding co-morbidities can all be informed by HF/E. Devices will need to be designed for these ageing users, and a better understanding of care delivery in the home will be beneficial. Similarly, cultural changes will require considerations not just of language in the design of work, but also more varied norms, expectations and standards. Again, HF/E techniques can explore and assist in the design of approaches to these challenges that are more likely to be successful. Ignoring them, or not designing for the humans at the centre of the system, is likely to lead to more expense, illness, and accidental harm.

The Educational Landscape for HF/E in Health and Social Care

In this book we have described HF/E as both a science and a practice. The science of HF/E studies the ways in which people interact with the systems in which they work. The knowledge gained through the science (and the methodologies, methods and tools so developed) are applied in practice with the twin aims of optimising system performance and improving human well-being. Implicit in this definition is the fact that HF/E is a profession; HF/E professionals will have undergone advanced training, usually to postgraduate level, and will have had many years of experience, often under the mentorship of more experienced colleagues. Usually, they will also have demonstrated their competency by going through a professional accreditation process with their relevant national professional body, such as the CIEHF in the UK. In short, the route to recognition as an HF/E professional is similar in process to that of a clinician. Despite what is inferred by the proliferation of HF/E short courses (including 'Masterclasses'), competency is not something that can be delivered as a one-off bolt-on. This is perhaps one of the main messages around HF/E education. In the same way that we would encourage human factors integration within an organisation, we would also encourage its long-term sustainability by ensuring an education and training strand forms part of that integration strategy.

If you are personally involved in providing HF/E education and training, it is as important as in any other area of your work that you consider your scope of practice. Most professional education bodies describe what might be called the 'dimensions' of teaching practice. These include things like *activities* (the things educators do), the *knowledge* they use in doing these activities and the *values* that inform their work. A lot of it is about pedagogy, but the rest is about quality assuring and enhancing your activity and the subject-specific knowledge. But just how much do you need to know? Interestingly, if you look across the pedagogical literature, the contribution of subject-specific knowledge wasn't really considered until the 1990s – it was assumed that you needed to be a subject matter expert to teach. Much more of the research was about the importance of 'learning about learning'. However, if we look at what really goes on in educational establishments across the world (so, educational work-as-done) we can see that very effective teaching is frequently delivered by teachers who are barely a few steps ahead of the learners. There is also quite a bit of evidence that suggests there is real value in being taught by a non-expert – they are not too far beyond the learners, and the struggles they had with the material are fresher in their minds than is the case with experts.

So are we saying that teaching by non-experts goes well most of the time? That sounds like a good argument for a bit of Safety-II. In formal education programmes, such as our undergraduate healthcare programmes, we can see that we deliver successful outcomes most of the time, despite not all teachers being experts. What supports this good performance? There are probably several main factors, the first being some pedagogical insight and understanding. Other factors include:

- First, having a strategy for self-diagnosis and evaluation of the subject matter knowledge you do have.
- Second, effective non-experts do have a high-level understanding of the subject, so they are able to recognise the key concepts and the relationships between them. As a side note, one of the problems that non-technical skills trainers often have is that they do not have sufficient understanding of the breadth of the HF/E discipline.
- Third, non-experts have somewhere to go to when they are not sure. They have support networks that include access (however informal) to people with more expertise. In that way, they can sense-check their teaching.

Probably the most important take home message from this is the importance of building networks and being able to recognise high-quality education options to support your own continuing professional development (CPD). In the UK, there are several such options, and the CIEHF-accredited Healthcare Learning Pathway and the training associated with the NHS England Patient Safety Syllabus are described below.

NHS England National Patient Safety Syllabus

The NHS England Patient Safety Syllabus is multi-professional and NHS-wide. The associated curriculum is a work in progress but aims to support the development of training in fundamentals of safety for all staff. In addition, it covers advanced training for staff with additional safety responsibilities, such as patient safety specialists. Patient safety specialists are envisaged as providing 'dynamic safety leadership' within their organisations. It is a requirement for all organisations to appoint at least one such person. There are five domains in the syllabus: (1) Systems approach to safety; (2) Learning from incidents; (3) Human factors, human performance and safety management; (4) Creating safe systems; and (5) Being sure about safety. There are different levels of depth and breadth of knowledge associated with different roles. An introductory e-learning module is available to all staff in the NHS in England, while in-depth training consisting of both e-learning as well as in-person days is available to the smaller group of designated patient safety specialists. One of the criticisms in the way the patient safety syllabus is made available is the narrow focus on job title (patient safety specialist) rather than competency required for the job. In response, a national community of practice and network of patient safety practitioners, most of whom are not designated patient safety specialists, has developed to provide a safe space for shared learning and peer support.

CIEHF-Accredited Healthcare Learning Pathway

The CIEHF Healthcare Learning Pathway is one of several industry-specific Learning Pathways offered by CIEHF. Initially developed as a partnership between CIEHF, Loughborough University, Robert Gordon University, NHS Education for Scotland, Human Factors Everywhere Ltd and Health Education England, the Healthcare Learning Pathway is currently offered by Loughborough University. It provides a route to professional recognition as a Technical Specialist (Healthcare) with CIEHF. There are three levels, with Level 1 being the same as for the Patient Safety Syllabus (Health Education England chose to adopt this package for its own Level 1 training). Level 2 comprises nine courses, which address the following topics: (1) Systems; (2) Task analysis; (3) Teamwork, non-technical skills and leadership; (4) Procedures; (5) Risk analysis and resilience; (6) Incident investigation; (7) Medical devices and digital interfaces; (8) Communicating HF/E; and (9) Physical environment.

These modules are delivered through a mix of synchronous and asynchronous online activities. Level 3 offers the opportunity for mentorship. Over the course of (typically) one year, participants will be supported in HF/E activities in their own workplace and are guided to present these in the form of logbook entries for subsequent assessment for Technical Membership.

Achieving Sustainable Change

During the COVID-19 pandemic, CIEHF published a guidance document on Achieving Sustainable Change: Capturing Learning from COVID-19 (CIEHF, 2020). This guidance describes how systems thinking and organisational learning can contribute to sustainable change following the pandemic. It is fitting to conclude this book with this ambition. We have presented HF/E as a scientific discipline and a professional practice that emphasises systems thinking, and helps embrace the messiness of the complex systems that we find in health and social care. HF/E supports effective analysis and design with scientific and evidenced-based methods, considering principles of equality, diversity and inclusion, to support usability, accessibility, performance and safety.

From here on, it is over to you, the HF/E practitioner, the enthusiast, and the champion for HF/E in your organisations. Successful adoption of HF/E in practice is best regarded as a journey. The journey is easier when you network and share learning and experiences with others. Professional membership bodies, such as the Chartered Institute of Ergonomics and Human Factors in the UK, provide vibrant communities of practice, where you can continue your HF/E journey in many different ways. You can share and discuss with peers, you can seek out experts, and you can continue your own guided learning by seeking professional accreditation. The CIEHF website offers a wealth of resources, including webinars and downloadable guidance documents to support you with your HF/E journey and integration of HF/E in your organisation (CIEHF, 2024).

It is important that we, as the HF/E community, share our stories and insights in order to help us develop a compelling case for HF/E in achieving sustainable change in health and social care. We invite you on this journey and to help us learn from one another.

References

CIEHF. 2020. *Achieving Sustainable Change*. https://ergonomics.org.uk/resource/achieving-sustainable-change.html
CIEHF. 2021. *Human Factors in Healthcare AI*. https://ergonomics.org.uk/resource/human-factors-in-healthcare-ai.html
CIEHF. 2024. *Homepage*. https://ergonomics.org.uk/

Index

A

Accidents 83, 141, 143, 144–145, 177
Accountability 34, 147–148; see also Blame
ACTA see Applied Cognitive Task Analysis
Adverse events 33, 130–132, 134–135, 143
Affordances 117–118, 123–124
Anthropometric data 94–95
Applied Cognitive Task Analysis (ACTA) 164
Artificial Intelligence (AI) 135–136, 180–181
Attention 78, 83, 101–103, 107–108
Auditory processing 101–103

B

Behaviour 17, 22–23, 79–80, 87, 97, 174
    approaches, behavioural 17, 22, 79, 87, 119
    change, behavioural 51–52, 87, 174
    behavioural marker systems 80–81
Bias 51, 135–136, 147, 180
Blame 23, 25–26, 34, 77, 87, 132, 142, 148; see also Accountability, Culture
    fear of 25–26
    reduction of 24, 142
Blood test 6–8, 99–100
Burnout 27, 33, 77, 130–133

C

Capability-demand theory 57–58, 67–69
Care, delivery of 10, 73, 76, 78, 156–157
Chartered Institute of Ergonomics and Human Factors (CIEHF) 125, 144, 154, 161–163, 170, 181–184
    CIEHF Healthcare Learning Pathway 183
    competencies 16, 35, 53–54, 72–73, 88–89, 110–111, 126, 137, 150, 165, 176
    sustainable change 144–146
CIEHF see Chartered Institute of Ergonomics and Human Factors

Climate assessment tools/safety culture 24–26
Co-design 14, 63, 99, 155
Cognition 75, 80, 82–86, 101–102
Cognitive performance 57, 97, 105–107; see also cognitive tasks
Communication 77–80, 85–86, 101–103, 132
Consultation 69, 160–162
Controls 113–118, 124–125
COVID-19 pandemic 101, 144, 154, 155–156, 184
    design of delivery system 123–125
Crew resource management (CRM) 80, 87
CRM see Crew resource management
Culture
    blame 23, 77, 132, 142, 148
    change in 21–23, 77
    development 22–23
    core principle of 22
    layers 22–23
    practical culture 22–23
    safety culture 20–29, 33–34, 131, 175

D

Decision making 82–86, 107–109
    Distributed cognition (DC) 85–86
    Distributed Cognition for Teamwork (DiCoT) 86
    shared 97
    recognition–primed decision (RPD) model 85
Design
    co-design see co-design.
    environment 91–95, 105–110
    equipment 55, 60, 93–96
    inclusive 65–69
    Inclusive Design Toolkit 69

Index

    organisational processes 5, 19–20, 33, 118–119
    software 118–119
    systems 3–5, 20, 113–126, 179–180
    tasks 37–54
    universal design principles 68–69
    user-centred 14, 113–114, 124–125
    workplace 57, 91–93
Deviations 67, 146
Dialogue 79, 85, 143
Distributed cognition (DC) 85–86
Distributed Situation Awareness (DSA) 83–84
Double loop 20
DSA *see* Distributed Situation Awareness

E

Education 181–183
    CIEHF Healthcare Learning Pathway 183
Environment 91–111
    acoustic environment 101–103
    change to 22, 71
    clinical 10, 19, 23, 62, 91, 105
    healthcare 107–109
    human-centred approach 109–110
    layout of 96–100
    non-clinical 181
    lighting of 101, 103–105
    physical 17, 57, 73, 91–96
    temperature 105–107
Emergency care 77–78, 84
    employee
    illness, injury 3, 13, 93–95, 104, 107, 131
    performance 3–4, 37, 47, 59, 96–97, 129, 132
    training 4, 26, 119, 176
    well-being 8, 10–11, 14, 27, 59, 63–64, 93, 101, 104–105, 129–131, 133, 183
Equality, diversity and inclusion (EDI) 153–165
    international standards 163–165
    health disparities 156–157
    protected characteristics 157–159
    systems approach 159–160
Error 47–50, 82–83, 113–114, 122–124, 164; *see also* Human error
EUROCONTROL Health and Social Care Safety Culture Discussion Cards 29–31

Events *see* Adverse events, incidents
Exclusion 67, 155–156

F

Failure modes and effects analysis (FMEA) 45
Fatigue 6, 13, 18, 27, 31, 50, 57–59, 63–64, 65, 77, 97, 107, 131–132, 171
Feedback 116–117, 123, 132, 142, 146

H

Handovers 27, 78
Hazards 47, 52, 67, 94, 141, 175
Hazard and Operability Studies (HAZOP) 67
Health and Social Care Safety Culture Discussion Cards 29–31
Healthcare Quality Improvement Partnership (HQIP) 156
Health disparities 156–157
Health Services Safety Investigations Body (HSSIB) 142
Heuristics 51, 118–119, 169
Hierarchical task analysis (HTA) 40–44, 99, 119
HQIP *see* Healthcare Quality Improvement Partnership
HSSIB *see* Health Services Safety Investigations Body
Hub and spoke model 174
Human-centred approach 109–110, 167–169
Human-centred system 181
Human Factors/ergonomics
    definition 2–3
    twin aims of 3–4, 129
    integration of 167–176
    methods 13–15
Human factors integration (HFI) 167–176
Human failure analysis 45–47
Human reliability analysis 38, 45, 50–51

I

Incidents 141; *see also* Accidents, Patient Safety Incident Response Framework (PSIRF)
Reporting 141–143
Illness 131–132
Improvement interventions 10–12, 64, 114, 125, 132–135

Index

Injuries 93–94
Input-process-output model 81
Integration of Human Factors 167–176
Integrated Workload Scale (IWS) 62
International Organization for Standardization (ISO) 120–122, 163, 167
Intervention selection 51–52
Involvement 29, 147–148, 161–164
ISO see International Organization for Standardization
IWS see Integrated Workload Scale

J

Just culture 29, 34

K

Kirwan, Barry 174

L

Leadership 32, 80, 162–163
Learning 139–150
Learning incidents (LFI) 140
Learning from Patient Safety Events service (LfPSE) 142
Lighting 101, 103–106
Link analysis 98–100
Local rationality 34, 143

M

Manchester Patient Safety Assessment Framework (MaPSaF) 27
Mapping workshops 69–70
Maturity axis 28
Metacognition 82
MBRRACE-UK reports 156–157
Measurement futures 136
Medications 38, 47, 67, 93, 104, 159–160, 173; see also pharmacy
Medical devices 113–126
Morecambe Bay NHS Foundation Trust 23

N

NASA see National Aeronautics and Space Administration
NASA-TLX see National Aeronautics and Space Administration Task Load Index

National Aeronautics and Space Administration (NASA) 141
National Aeronautics and Space Administration Task Load Index (NASA-TLX) 62
National Reporting and Learning System (NRLS) 141
NHS England National Patient Safety Syllabus 183
NHS Health Check 19, 29–31
Noise 102–103, 107–109
Non-technical skills (NTS) 80–81
NRLS see National Reporting and Learning System

O

Occupational health 64, 173
Onion model 22
Organisational culture see organisations
Organisations 17–35
    culture of 18–20, 31–33
    dimensions 29
    influences 19
    measuring performance 27–28
    NHS Health Check 19
    performance-influencing factors 30–33, 47–51, 58–64
    processes, organisation 5, 19–20, 33, 118–119
    resilience 33–34
Outcomes 129–137
    different types of 130–131
    patient 130–131, 149, 156–157
    measures and monitoring 133–135
    system and well-being outcomes 131–133

P

Participation 160–162
Patient Safety 19, 29, 83, 130, 141–149
    Patient Safety Incident Response Framework (PSIRF) 139, 142, 146–149
    four pillars of 148–149
    capability-demand theory 58
    designing for inclusion 66
    anthropometric measurements 66
    HAZOP 67
    inadvertent exclusion 67

designing to meet human characteristic
defining user capabilities 65–66
users 65, 114–115
mapping workshops 69–70
performance-influencing factors (PIFs) 58–64
personas 71
People 55–73, 91; see also employees
capabilities 55–56
Perception 101–108
Performance 112, 129–137, 143–146; see also Performance-influencing factors
environment, influenced by 103–107
measuring 27–28
tasks 37–38
Performance-influencing factors (PIFs) 18, 37, 45, 47–51, 58–64
common workload assessment methods 61–62
fatigue 63–64
pharmacists 31
stress 62–63
workload 58–60
Personas 71, 121
Person-centred care 157
Pharmacy 10, 31, 33, 67
Policies and procedures 19–20, 119–122
standardising 20
Procurement 55, 93–95, 121–122, 170–173
Protected characteristics 158–159
Psychological factors 27, 59, 62–64, 82–86; see also well-being
Performance-shaping factors (PSF) see Performance-influencing factors (PIFs)

Q

Quality improvement (QI) 13, 37
Quantitative versus qualitative data 134–135

R

Randomised control trials 134–135
Rapid Entire Body Assessment (REBA) 96–98
RawTLX 62
Recognition-primed decision (RPD) model 85
Resilience 33–34, 63, 144–145
organisational 33–34

Responsibility 29, 34, 147–148
Reporting systems 27, 141–143
Resources, availability 29, 59, 131, 133
Risk management 51–53, 142–143
Root cause analysis (RCA) 141–142, 146

S

Safety-I and Safety-II 145
Safety climate 27
Safety culture 20–27, 30–31, 33–34, 175
challenges of 20
characteristics 33
climate assessment tools 24–26
maturity axis 28
SEIPS see Systems Engineering Initiative for Patient Safety
Sensory deficits 103–104
Sepsis bundle elements of 6
Serious Incident Framework (SIF) 146–147
Service improvement see Quality improvement
Service, review 19
Seven Cs Model 79
SHERPA see Systematic Human Error Reduction and Prediction Approach
Signal detection theory 108
Situation awareness (SA) 82–84
advantage of 82
Distributed Situation Awareness model 83–84
examples of 83
healthcare setting 84
Staffing levels 31, 33, 40, 49–50, 52, 131–132
Standardisation 20
Stress 6, 8, 27, 33, 50, 57, 59, 61–63, 65, 72, 77, 97, 101, 106, 109–110, 118, 130, 131, 132, 133; see also fatigue, burnout
Subjective Workload Assessment Technique (SWAT) 61–62
SWAT see Subjective Workload Assessment Technique
Systematic Human Error Reduction and Prediction Approach (SHERPA) 45–47, 58
credible error 46
human error taxonomy 46
performance-influencing factors 47–50

Systems
   clinical 84
   coupled 11
   sociotechnical 3, 13, 114, 127, 153, 159
   thinking 15–16, 21, 34, 150, 179, 184
Systems approach 4–5, 20–21, 159–160
Systems Engineering Initiative for Patient Safety (SEIPS) 5–6, 129–133

T

Tasks
   analysis 38, 40–45, 88
   clinical 3, 40–44, 82–83
   cognitive 39, 82–86
   design of 37–38
   hierarchical task analysis 40–45, 99
   human capabilities 55–56
   human reliability analysis 38, 45–51
   implementation and monitoring 53
   increase in 57
   intervention selection 51–52
   medicines reconciliation 38
   selection of 39–40, 108
   types 39
   vulnerabilities 37, 45–51
Task analysis (TA) *see* tasks, analysis
Task load index *see* NASA-TLX
Teams 76–88, 144, 161, 173–174
   multi-professional 76–77
Teamwork and non-technical skills 75–89; *see also* teams
   activities 78
   decision-making models 85–86
   delivery 86
   in health and social care 77–79
   non-technical skills 80–81
   'Seven Cs' model 79
   situation awareness 82–84
   systems-thinking principles for 76–77
   TeamSTEPPS 80
   words of caution 86–88

Technology 9, 113–126, 170–171, 180–181
   automation 117
   controls 115–116
   display 116
   functionality 116–117
   regulation of 120–122
Temperature 105–107
   regulation of 105–106
Tools 9, 113–126
   design of delivery system 123–124
   controls 115–116
   concept of affordances 117–118
   controls 115–116
   decision-making failure 114
   displays 116
   functionality 116–117
   heuristics 118–119
   instructions and training 119–122
   steps for medical devices 120–122
   users 114–115
Trade-offs 11, 31, 129, 143, 146, 179
Training 119–122, 176, 182–183; *see also* Employee

U

Usability 113–115, 118–120, 122, 163, 171; *see also* Design, user-centred
Users 65–71, 114–115, 121
Universal design principles 68–69

W

Well-being 8, 10–11, 14, 27, 59, 63–64, 93, 101, 104–110, 129–131, 133, 163, 183
Work
   as-imagined 33–34, 143
   as-done 33–34, 143
Workarounds 12, 91, 179
Work context 17, 29–31, 58–59, 86–87, 115–116, 171
Workload 50, 58–62, 77, 98–99, 114, 117
   assessment of 62